Urog

Evide... Based

Clinical Practice

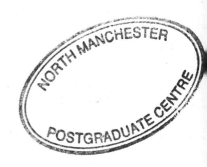

Urogynecology: Evidence-Based Clinical Practice

Kate H. Moore

With 61 Figures

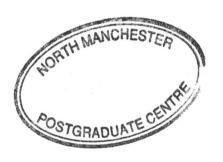

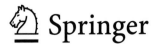 Springer

Kate H. Moore, MBBS, FRCOG, FRANZCOG, MD, CU
Associate Professor
Department of Urogynaecology
The Pelvic Floor Unit
St George Hospital
University of New South Wales
Sydney
Australia

Cover illustration: Fig. 4.12: Urine trapping in a dependant cystocycle after voiding.

British Library Cataloguing in Publication Data
Moore, Kate H.
   Urogynecology in clinical practice
   1. Urogynecology   2. Urodynamics   3. Urinary incontinence   4. Urinary
incontinence – Treatment   5. Women – Diseases – Treatment
   I. Title
   616.6′0082

ISBN-10: 1-84628-164-4   e-ISBN 1-84628-165-2   Printed on acid-free paper
ISBN-13: 978-1-84628-164-8

Printed in the United States of America   (EB/BP)

9 8 7 6 5 4 3 2 1

Springer Science+Business Media
springer.com

Foreword
Urogynaecology—Evidenced Based Clinical Practice

It is just over twenty years since Urogynaecology achieved international recognition as a Subspeciality of Gynaecology. During that time urogynaecology has attracted a burgeoning interest, as evidenced by the large number of doctors and nurses who have taken up and become expert in this field, and the extensive outpouring of original and sterling research accompanied by significant sophistication in studies and their evaluation; all gratefully acknowledged by the many women all over the world whose lives have been made miserable by the common and indifferently treated conditions of incontinence, urinary infection and prolapse.

These topics represent the tip of the Urogynaecological iceberg, with a range and spectrum of maladies united often by the common thread of a damaged pelvic floor. We no longer use the historical and anatomical divisions of pelvic floor function, but instead take a holistic view of the pelvic floor as one physiological unit whose damage leads to disordered function in all three pelvic compartments. No speciality gives a better example of interdisciplinary collaboration than Urogynaecology, with Urologists, Colo-rectal surgeons and Gynaecologists working in close co-operation—a relationship which has lead to cross fertilization between the specialties in research and clinical practice.

This book for Obstetricians and Gynaecologists in training is written by Kate Moore, an internationally known and respected Urogynaecologist, who has, herself, made significant contributions to both research and clinical practice in Urogynaecology.

This book is unique in its approach, not just to Urogynaecology but to the correct way of managing a patient where the patient's ease and access to information is regarded as being as important as the evaluation and successful treatment of her condition. The author recognises and practises the cardinal principles of medicine in the twenty first century—that medicine should be evidence-based, with emphasis on standardised, subjective and objective outcome measures and the need to rely on a multi-disciplinary team to give the best clinical outcome.

Patients, colleagues and students will be grateful to Kate Moore for the clarity, wide intellectual scope and clinical expertise which this book achieves.

Preface

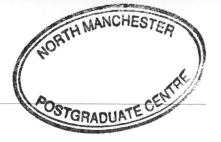

This textbook aims to serve the needs of the pre-membership registrar/resident medical officer/senior house officer who has been attached to a urogynecology department, who needs a clear "how to do it" text. It is hoped that it will also be useful to consultant gynecologists, who received no formal urogynecological training during their pre-membership years, and would like a quick practical update.

The prevalence of urinary incontinence and prolapse is increasing in the Western world as the population becomes more elderly. Thus there is increasing need for knowledge about this subject.

Although there are several recent large costly authoritative texts that cover the whole subject in depth, these are most suited to postmembership registrars in subspecialty training, or gynecologists who have already developed a major interest in the subject. There are few small "pocket-sized" books that give the practical elements of the subject, based upon current evidence, but without lengthy discussion of the current controversies in the area (which are numerous). Small books are available about urodynamic testing, but feature a heavy emphasis upon the voiding phase that is so important for male incontinence.

This text assumes a basic undergraduate knowledge of the difference between stress incontinence and urge incontinence, eg incontinence arising from a weak urethral sphincter or an overactive detrusor muscle. Because practical matters are emphasized, discussion of the epidemiology or etiology of conditions is very brief.

The management of stress incontinence has changed radically in the last decade, and surgery for prolapse has also evolved considerably. For many years, fecal incontinence and obstructed defecation were considered to be completely separate subjects, but are now known to interrelate with many urogynecological disorders. Obstetrician gynecologists have become more aware that labor ward practices have an impact upon the pelvic floor. Hence knowledge of these subjects is now a vital part of urogynecology.

In this text, success rates are given according to standardized outcome measures where possible, as recommended by the

International Continence Society. The recommendations of the Cochrane Collaboration on Urinary Incontinence and the World Health Organization Consensus Conferences on Incontinence are also incorporated.

ACKNOWLEDGEMENTS
Sincere thanks to Carol Bagshaw for manuscript preparation, to Albert Lun of Medical Illustrations Department of St. George Hospital for graphic design, to all the staff of the Pelvic Floor Unit and to Ross Mullane.

Contents

Chapter 1
Taking the History

This chapter deals first with incontinence/voiding dysfunction, then prolapse and fecal incontinence. Detailed history-taking for bacterial cystitis and interstitial cystitis are included in the relevant chapters, but the basic features are given here.

Many urogynecology patients have multiple symptoms, for example, mixed stress and urge leak along with prolapse, or postoperative voiding difficulty with recurrent cystitis and dyspareunia. It is important to untangle or dissect the different problems and then tackle them one by one (although the total picture must fit together at the end).

To help you manage the patient, ask, "What is your main problem. What bothers you the most?" Only after you have sorted this question out fully, should a systematic review be undertaken. Let the patient tell you her story.

HISTORY TAKING FOR INCONTINENT WOMEN

Incontinence Symptoms
Stress incontinence (leakage with cough, sneeze, lifting heavy objects; see Figure 1.1A).

Note that stress incontinence is a symptom.

Stress incontinence is a physical sign (see Chapter 2).

Urodynamic stress incontinence means that on urodynamic testing the patient leaks with a rise in intra-abdominal pressure, in the absence of a detrusor contraction (see Figure 1.1B and Chapter 4).

Urge incontinence (leakage with the desperate desire to void) is a symptoms that is difficult to elicit on physical examination (see Chapter 2).

On urodynamic testing, if the patient leaks when a detrusor contraction occurs, associated with the symptom of urgency, the condition is termed detrusor overactivity (see Chapter 4).

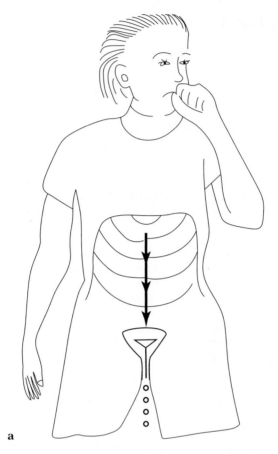

a

FIGURE 1.1. **(a)** Stress incontinence, leakage associated with raised intra-abdominal pressure.

Many patients will have mixed stress and urge incontinence, but can tell you which one bothers them the most, or makes them leak the most.

Take the time to ask the patient, because this guides initial therapy, and helps you to interpret urodynamic tests.

Nonincontinent Symptoms of Storage Disorders:
Frequency, Urgency, Nocturia

Frequency of micturition is defined as eight or more voids per day.

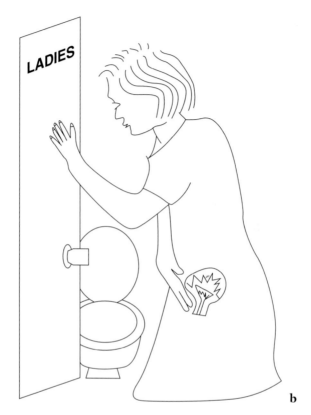

b

FIGURE 1.1. **(b)** Urge incontinence, leakage associated with a detrusor contraction.

The normal adult with an average fluid intake of 1.5–2 liters per day will void 5–6 times per day.

If a woman has increased frequency, ask whether she voids "just in case": before going shopping and so on, because many women with stress incontinence do this to avoid having a full bladder when they lift shopping bags and the like. The difference is important.

The woman with an overactive detrusor muscle will rush to the toilet frequently because she has an urgent desire to void, caused by the bladder spasm, and she is afraid she will leak if she does not make the toilet on time. The urgent desire to void for fear of leakage is defined as "urgency".

Nocturia is defined as the regular need to pass urine once or more per night in women aged 60 or less. One episode of nocturia is allowed per decade thereafter, eg twice per night in the seventy-year old is not considered abnormal (as renal perfusion in the elderly improves at night when the patient lies down and blood flow to the kidneys increases).

The overactive bladder (OAB) is a clinical syndrome, not a urodynamic diagnosis. It comprises frequency, urgency, nocturia, with or without urge incontinence (in the absence of bacterial cystitis or hematuria). It was defined by the International Continence Society in order to help general practitioners to identify patients likely to have detrusor overactivity, so that they could be treated in the general practice setting without recourse to urodynamic testing.

THE FREQUENCY VOLUME CHART (FVC)

This chart (Figure 1.2) is especially helpful in assessing whether the patient suffers from daytime frequency or nocturia, and how much urine she generally can store (her functional bladder capacity). The average patient has difficulty remembering exactly how often she voids, and of course has no idea of the volume she can store.

Most urogynecologists send out a blank FVC to patients prior to the first visit, so she can complete it before the first visit. See Chapter 5 (Outcome Measures) for more detail. This is a crucial part of starting bladder training for patients with overactive bladder (see Chapter 7).

Other Types of Leakage

These may denote a more complex situation.

Leakage when rising from the sitting position can be due to stress incontinence (relative rise in abdominal pressure when standing) or due to urge incontinence (gravitational receptors in the wall of the bladder trigger a detrusor contraction upon standing).

"Leakage without warning" is a nonspecific but important symptom. It may indicate detrusor overactivity, when a patient reaches her threshold bladder volume triggering a detrusor contraction. It may also indicate stress incontinence that the patient cannot verbalize; eg, she leaks with the slightest movement.

Leakage when arising from bed at night to go to the toilet is also nonspecific but important. Nocturia usually is associated with an overactive bladder. However, some patients with

Please fill in this chart before coming to the Unit; it gives your doctor important information and can help you to understand your condition.

Please fill in the <u>approximate time</u> and <u>amount</u> of how much fluid you drink, as illustrated in the example below.

Please fill in the <u>correct time</u> and <u>amount</u> of how much water (urine) you passed: either millilitres or ounces. Please mark with a star * when you leak/when pad is damp. Fill in the chart for 3 days (e.g. 3 x 24 hours = 72 hours) in a row.

Date/Time	Fluids taken in	Amount of urine passed mls or ounces	*= wet	Date/Time	Fluids taken in	Amount of urine passed mls or ounces	*= wet
EXAMPLE / ILLUSTRATION :				1.7.05			
1.6.99 2AM	—	150 mls		0720		550 ml	*
7 AM	—	250 mls	*	0730	Cup Orange		
8AM	Mug coffee	—		0745	Cup tea		
8.20	—	60 mls	*	0830		160 ml	
9.30	Cup orange	—		1015	Cup Coffee		
10.00	—	100 mls		1030	Cup Coffee		
12.00	2 mugs coffee	—		1130		380 ml	*
14.00		360 mls	*	1245	Glass Water		
AND	SO ON FOR 3 DAYS			2pm		260 ml	
				400	Cup of tea		
30.6.05				450		180 ml	
07/5		580 ml	*	6pm	Soda Water		
0730	Cup Orange			730		310 ml	
0745	Cup tea			930	Cup of Tea		
0830		190 ml		1015		230 ml	
10am	Cup tea			2.7.05			
1015		350 ml		715		590 ml	*
12	Glass water			730	Cup Orange		
330		410 ml	*	745	Cup tea	175 ml	
400	Cup tea			0830		175 ml	
450		170 ml		10am	Cup tea		
6pm	Glass beer			11am	Cup tea		
730		360	*	1245		420 ml	*
945	Cup tea						
1015		200					

FIGURE 1.2. Frequency Volume Chart, showing a patient with good bladder volumes, adequate fluid intake, and typical stress leak. Note the "just in case" voiding before going to work (08:30) and coming home (4:50 PM) in the train.

a very weak sphincter and other causes for nocturia (such as night sweats, obstructive sleep apnea, or a snoring husband) may leak as soon as they get up to go to the toilet.

Leakage during intercourse is seldom volunteered. Ask this question tactfully. Coital incontinence that occurs during penetration is most likely due to stress incontinence, whereas leakage during orgasm is more likely due to detrusor overactivity.

HOW BAD IS THE PROBLEM?

Some patients use only a damp pantyliner once daily, but their mother was grossly incontinent in her old age and they do not wish to become like her. Other patients use many large pads fully soaked per day but have put up with it for years owing to embarrassment. It is important to assess severity because evidence indicates that mild incontinence is more readily cured by conservative measures. Severe stress incontinence is more likely to need surgery. Severe urge incontinence is logically more likely to require anticholinergic drugs.

Many Units now quantitate the severity of leakage by asking three standardized questions, which have a set range of answers, in a format defined by the World Health Organization. For illustration see Chapter 5, but the questions are as follows.

- How often do you leak urine? (All the time, daily, two to three times weekly, weekly, or less)
- How much urine do you leak? (A little bit, a moderate amount, a large amount)
- How much does it affect your daily life? (On a scale of 1 to 10)

HISTORY TAKING FOR VOIDING DIFFICULTY

Although difficulty in emptying the bladder as a primary complaint occurs in only about 4% of females presenting with lower urinary tract symptoms, voiding difficulty does commonly accompany other urogynecological problems such as prolapse, and can be a lifelong problem in women who have previously had continence surgery.

The classic complaints are:

- Needing to strain to void, eg the urine does not come away without a Valsalva strain to start the flow (this is never normal).
- The flow is intermittent: "stop—start".

■ The flow is prolonged (the patient takes much longer to void than her friends or others in a public bathroom at the movies).

■ Post-void dribble: the patient gets up from the toilet thinking she is empty but urine trickles out as she walks away.

■ Need to revoid: the patient gets up from the toilet thinking she has finished but has to go back to the toilet within a few minutes.

■ Recurrent episodes of bacterial cystitis.

All such patients need free uroflowmetry with post-void residual, and voiding cystometry if these are abnormal (see Chapter 4).

The underlying causes may be:

Prolapse with urine trapping
Post-surgical urethral obstruction
Underactive detrusor (more common in the older woman)
Urethral diverticulum

HISTORY TAKING FOR PROLAPSE

"Something coming down in the vagina" is the classic statement. The patient may have a wide range of severity of symptoms. It is important to define how badly she is affected.

■ In mild cases, she may sometimes feel a lump the size of a small egg at the introitus when she is washing herself in the shower after standing up all day at work (not every day).

■ In more severe cases, she feels an obvious lump there every time she washes, and sometimes feels that there is a lump protruding when she sits down, so that she is uncomfortable. She may find the lump uncomfortable during intercourse, or too embarrassing so that she refuses to have intercourse.

■ In very severe cases, the lump is there in her underwear all the time, associated with a low backache or nagging discomfort.

■ In the worst-case scenario, the lump rubs on her underwear and causes staining either brown or red (due to dependant edema with trauma), and she may experience an unpleasant abdominal pain if there is a low-lying enterocele with traction on the nerves to the small bowel.

HISTORY TAKING FOR FECAL INCONTINENCE

Fecal incontinence is really the wrong term to use. We should be asking about anal incontinence, which includes incontinence to flatus and feces. Incontinence of flatus from the anus is very socially debilitating and should not be ignored.

Flatus incontinence is defined as regular passage of noisy or foul-smelling gas which the patient is attempting to inhibit, or which seeps out without any warning sensation. Even if this occurs once per month during an important business meeting, it can be disastrous.

Fecal incontinence is usually broken down into:
—Only when the stool is liquid (with diarrhea). Note whether patient has inflammatory bowel disease or malabsorption symptoms; treating the underlying disease may cure the problem.
—Incontinence when the stool is solid usually indicates a more severe problem and can have a devastating impact on the patient's life.

Assessing severity:
—Does the patient need to wear a pad for the leakage, or an anal plug (Figure 1.3)?
—Does the patient need to take constipating medicine to stop leakage of watery stool?
—Ask about fecal urgency, defined as unable to defer the call to stool for 15 minutes.

All these aspects of severity are included in the Wexner Score (see Chapter 5).

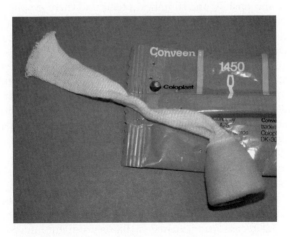

FIGURE 1.3. Anal plug.

SYMPTOMS OF OBSTRUCTIVE DEFECATION

■ Constipation, roughly defined as
   —Straining to pass hard stool
   —Not able to defecate daily (less than three motions per week)
■ Needing to digitate the vagina in order to expel hard stool
   —Often has to express the stool out manually
■ Post-defecation soiling with need to re-evacuate
   —Patient feels defecation is complete
   —Stands up to leave toilet
   —Feels stool coming onto underpants, or else
   —Feels more stool present in anal canal, has to sit down again

ASSESSING PREVIOUS SURGICAL HISTORY IN RELATION TO URINARY INCONTINENCE

If patient had previous continence surgery with persistent or recurrent leakage, there is a need to find out exactly what procedure she had (get notes or write to surgeon).

■ If previous anterior repair for incontinence
   —Failure is not surprising
■ If previous Pfannenstiel incision
   —Patient may not know whether this was Marshall–Marchetti procedure (failure is common) or a colposuspension (failure is less common; suspect detrusor overactivity)
■ If previous "sling", need to know whether this was
   —A true abdomino-vaginal sling
   —If so, whether autologous fascia (sheath or fascia lata from patient; failure uncommon)
   —Or whether synthetic mesh (may be undergoing rejection)
   —Or whether the "sling" was a Raz, Peyeyra, or Gittes type (failure very common; see Chapter 9)

If previous continence surgery failed, also check whether patient had **voiding difficulty**:

May have been sent home with supra-pubic catheter in situ
May have been trained to perform clean intermittent self-catheterization

These features mean that:

Patient could have sub-acute retention with overflow incontinence;

Further surgery in these cases is generally more likely to provoke voiding difficulty again.

HISTORY TAKING FOR DYSPAREUNIA
Any patient with urogynecology problems who also has dyspareunia needs this problem treated. The common features seen in urogynecology are as follows.

■ Post-operative scarring from overtight posterior repair
■ Post-operative scarring from overtight episiotomy repair
■ Post-colposuspension changes in the shape of the anterior vaginal wall
■ Atrophic vaginal changes (dryness, pruritis, coital discomfort)

General gynecological causes for superficial and deep dyspareunia should also be considered. For example, deep dyspareunia arising from endometriosis may co-exist, and laparoscopic treatment should be carried out (especially if surgery will be needed for the urogynecological complaint).

HISTORY TAKING FOR RECURRENT BACTERIAL CYSTITIS
This is covered in detail in Chapter 11, but the basics are as follows.

■ Has patient had >3 proven episodes of cystitis in last five years?
■ Has patient had renal ultrasound to exclude calculi?
■ Has patient had ultrasound to measure post-void residual?
■ Has patient had cystoscopy to investigate cystitis (need to get findings)?
■ Is cystitis often post-coital?
■ Are there post-menopausal atrophic vaginitis symptoms?
■ Has there been any haematuria, either during cystitis or at other times?

HISTORY TAKING FOR PAINFUL BLADDER SYNDROME/INTERSTITIAL CYSTITIS (IC)
This is covered in Chapter 12, but the basics include the following.

■ The main complaint is suprapubic pain.
　—Pain may be constant, or worse with a full bladder.

—Pain may be relieved by voiding.

—Pain may wax and wane over time.

■ Relentless frequency of micturition is typical, 10 to 20 times daily.

■ Severe nocturia is common but not present in all patients.

—Can be as severe as 5 to 10 nocturia episodes per night.

■ Bacterial cystitis should be excluded.

—The finding of proven recurrent bacterial cystitis generally precludes a diagnosis of IC.

HISTORY OF DRUG THERAPY THAT MAY FACILITATE URINARY INCONTINENCE

The most common culprit is the alpha adrenergic antagonist Prazocin (Minipress), which relaxes the innervation to the bladder neck and provokes stress incontinence. Always check exactly which antihypertensive the patient is using.

The next most common problem is use of diuretic therapy to treat hypertension. Although this may be good medical practice, it can be enough to tip the balance in a patient with a weak urethral sphincter, or an overactive bladder, into incontinence. Ask the patient's doctor whether another antihypertensive can be used.

A further common problem is the chronic dry cough seen with ACE inhibitors (especially Renitec, enlapril), which can provoke stress incontinence.

Many psychotropic drugs have anticholinergic effects that can precipitate chronic retention of urine with overflow incontinence. Lithium is a common culprit: it also is associated with increased thirst so patients accommodate increasingly large bladder volumes; eventually they cannot cope. The selective serotonin re-uptake inhibitors such as paroxetine, that also have some alpha adrenergic blockade effect, are also recently reported to cause chronic retention.

GENERAL ASSESSMENT OF THE PATIENT IN RELATION TO UROGYNECOLOGY

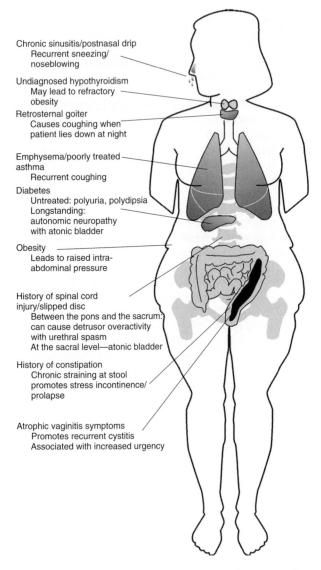

FIGURE 1.4. General factors contributing to the pathogenesis of incontinence or prolapse.

Chapter 2
Physical Examination

When examining a patient with urinary incontinence or prolapse, more care may be needed to be taken to avoid embarrassment than with the usual gynecology patient.

For example, a patient with menorrhagia is often fed up with her symptoms and just seeks your help to get rid of a practical problem that has little social stigma. On the other hand, a patient with incontinence often feels that she is "dirty" and "can't control herself." A patient with prolapse is often horrified about the lump appearing at her vaginal opening, and may have ceased intercourse because of embarrassment.

Therefore, always make sure that the patient's abdomen and genitalia are covered with a sheet, and only expose that part which you are about to examine. Establish a sympathetic rapport <u>before</u> you begin the examination.

EXAMINE THE ABDOMEN
Many patients attending the gynecologist for a first visit lie on the couch with their knees drawn up, assuming that only the vagina and pelvis will be examined. This is not appropriate in urogynecology: the abdomen must be examined first, so ask the patient to drop her knees down so that a relaxed abdominal exam can be performed.

Any mass that raises intra-abdominal pressure may cause incontinence.

- In our Unit, we see one to two patients per annum presenting with incontinence or urgency/frequency who in fact have an ovarian cyst (benign or malignant), or an enlarged uterus, that has previously been undetected.
- Also, patients may present with frequency and urgency but in fact have sub-acute retention, so it is important to percuss the abdomen to exclude an enlarged bladder. Shifting dullness

needs to be elicited if ascites is suspected, which may accompany an ovarian cancer that provokes stress incontinence.

■ Check the renal angles for tenderness, e.g. calculi.

INSPECT THE VULVA

First look for evidence of post-menopausal atrophy. Initially this appears as thin shiny glistening red epithelium, that appears fragile, rather than the healthy pink "skin" like appearance of the pre-menopausal women. Later changes include patchy whitish areas of cornification with some "cracks" or fissurelike lesions often between the labia majora and minora. In end stage, the labia minora may be fused at the midline. Urethral caruncle, a red rosebud appearance at the urethral meatus, also indicates estrogen deprivation (see Figure 2.1).

Do not be lulled into a sense of security because the patient is on systemic HRT. A percentage of these patients do not achieve

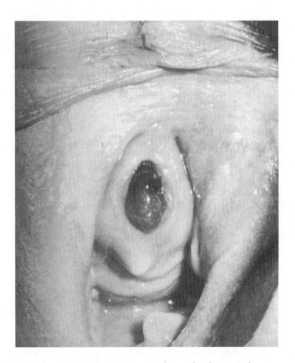

FIGURE 2.1. Classic atrophic vagina with urethral caruncle.

adequate blood levels in the vagina and vulva and may still get atrophic changes, which also affect the urethra.

Next, look at the introitus at rest, a cystocele or rectocele may be evident even without cough. Inspect the perineum for signs of post-obstetric perineal deficiency.

ELICIT A "STRESS LEAK"

Part the labia and ask the patient to cough. In order to save embarrassment, explain to the woman that you will place a piece of tissue/paper towel at the urethra, so that if she leaks, nothing will spill onto the linen. Patients are often terrified that they will leak urine in front of the doctor, yet this is exactly what we are trying to get them to do. You should have a tissue ready in any case, because a strong projectile spurt of urine may reach your clothing and embarrass the women even further (she will know if the spurt has been large enough to do this!).

Typically, a stress leak involves a short spurt of urine that occurs during the height of the cough effort. An urge leak typically occurs an instant after the cough, but a large prolonged urine leak is seen due to the detrusor contraction.

In practice, patients with urge incontinence will not get up onto your examining couch with a full bladder; they will always request to visit the toilet first.

Assess hypermobility of the anterior vaginal wall. When the patient coughs, there may not be a proper cystocele "bulge", but the whole anterior wall may move down with the cough.

SPECULUM EXAMINATION

Pass a Bi-valve Speculum

Always check that the cervix is healthy and take a Pap smear if due. As you withdraw the speculum check for normal vaginal epithelium as in any gynecological exam.

Pass a Sims Speculum

Traditional advice is to ask the patient to assume the left lateral position for a Sims speculum exam. In fact, if they are obese this may not be necessary; the bottom of the Sims may not hit the couch if the buttocks are sufficiently plump. If equipment is in short supply, the two leaves of a bivalve speculum can be unscrewed, and the anterior leaf used as a Sims speculum.

Cystocele (prolapse of the bladder into the vagina) and rectocele (prolapse of the rectum into the vagina) are traditionally graded (during Valsalva or cough) as the following.

- *Mild*: The prolapse descends more than halfway down the vagina but not to the introitus.
- *Moderate*: The prolapse descends to the level of the introitus.
- *Severe*: The prolapse descends well beyond the introitus and is outside of the vagina.
- Recently, the type of anterior prolapse has been divided into
  —Distension cystocele, resulting from overstretching in labor, or atrophic post-menopausal changes. The rugae have disappeared.
  —Displacement cystocele arises from tears in the lateral ligaments of the vagina. The vaginal rugae are usually still evident. If the lateral borders of the vagina are lifted with an open sponge forcep, the whole prolapse is easily replaced. This is more common in nullipara or women of low parity.
- Uterine descent follows the same classification, but if the majority of the organ is outside the vagina, the term procidentia is used.
- In highly parous women, the uterus may be well supported but the cervix may be very bulky and protuberant (worth noting when considering surgical options).
- Enterocele (prolapse of the small bowel into the vagina) is not a common major finding unless the patient has had a hysterectomy, when it is called a "vault enterocele" (the top of the post-hysterectomy vagina is called the vault). This prolapse is also graded mild/moderate/severe as above.

This "mild/moderate/severe" terminology has been used for many decades, and is called the Baden Walker system of classification.

POPQ SCORING SYSTEM OF PROLAPSE
Prior to the 1990s, the Baden Walker system of classification, as described above, was used, but it was realized that there is considerable subjectivity in defining "mild," moderate," and "severe" under this system. Therefore, urogynecologists devised a new system of measuring the degree of prolapse of the anterior and posterior walls of the vagina in centimeters, called Pelvic Organ Prolapse Quantification or POPQ (see Figure 2.2A).

First, the reference point of the introitus (the hymenal remnant) is taken as 0cm. Then using the normal vagina, a reference point of 3cm inside the introitus is called "−3cm", for both the anterior and posterior walls. When asking the patient to strain or cough, the distance that the cystocele or rectocele descends is measured.

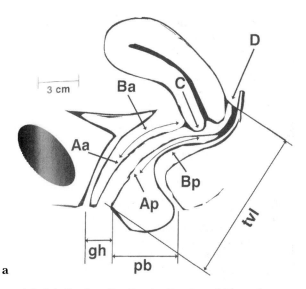

FIGURE 2.2. **(a)** Six sites (Aa, Ba, Ap, Bp, C, and D) used to quantitate POP.

When a normal woman coughs, the vaginal walls don't move, so the −3 point remains 3 cm inside the introitus. In a woman with cystocele, say eg that with cough the anterior wall (at the −3 point) protrudes out to 2 cm beyond the introitus. This is measured and recorded as +2 cm (meaning that the anterior wall at the reference point moves down by 5 cm with strain).

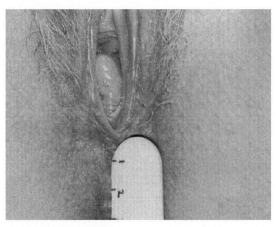

FIGURE 2.2. **(b)** Rectocele at the introitus with POPQ measuring device, perineum = 2.8 cm.

anterior wall	anterior wall	cervix or cuff
Aa	Ba	C
genital hiatus	perineal body	total vaginal length
gh	pb	tvl
posterior wall	posterior wall	posterior fornix
Ap	Bp	D

FIGURE 2.2. **(c)** POPQ definitions.

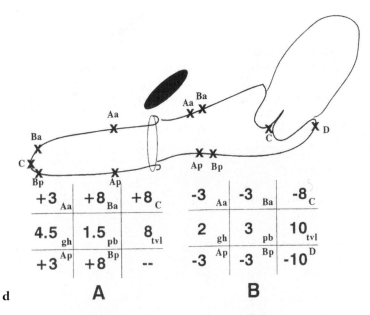

A			B		
+3 Aa	+8 Ba	+8 C	−3 Aa	−3 Ba	−8 C
4.5 gh	1.5 pb	8 tvl	2 gh	3 pb	10 tvl
+3 Ap	+8 Bp	--	−3 Ap	−3 Bp	−10 D

FIGURE 2.2. **(d)** Complete eversion of vagina POPQ. (A, C, and D are reprinted, with permission from Bump RC, Mattiasson A, Bo K et al (1996) The standardization of terminology of female pelvic organ prolapse and pelvic floor dysfunction. Am J Obstet Gynecol 175:10–1; Copyright 1996, Elsevier.)

Next the total vaginal length is measured, at the posterior fornix (as shown in Figure 2.2A) at Point D. Then the width of the perineal body is measured as shown in Figure 2.2B, from the fourchette to the mid-anal opening. The length of the genital hiatus, from the lower margin of the urethra to the inner aspect of the fourchette, is also measured.

These dimensions are recorded in the grid shown in Figure 2.2C.

Although the POPQ system may seem a little cumbersome to begin with, it is easy to pick up after a few practice attempts. Over the next decade, most gynecologists and all urogynecologists will inevitably take it up, because it is objective and allows for scientific research as to the outcome of prolapse surgery that has never been possible before (as shown in Chapter 9). The normal values, with an example of complete vault eversion, are shown in Figure 2.2D.

Perform a Bimanual Examination

Again, examine for pelvic masses that may press on the bladder to cause frequency, urgency, or incontinence. If a patient with incontinence comes to surgery, any other gynecological disorders such as menorrhagia with a large fibroid uterus, or ovarian cysts etc should be corrected at the same time; hence the term "urogynecology".

At the time of bimanual exam, if patient has had colposuspension, put the fingers into the retropubic space to feel for the typical "dimples" of the vagina adherent to the back of the pubic bone. If they are "rock solid" behind the bone, the operation is probably still anatomically intact. If not, the sutures may have come loose.

Also, palpate the urethra to feel for a cystic swelling, suggesting a urethral diverticulum.

ASSESS THE PELVIC FLOOR MUSCLE CONTRACTION STRENGTH—OXFORD SCORE

Several studies have shown that when asked to contract their pelvic floor muscles during examination, about 50 to 60% of women will mistakenly contract their gluteal muscles (lifting their buttocks off the couch slightly), or contract their abdominal muscles (which increases the intra-abdominal pressure, the opposite of what is needed).

It is important to place one finger partly in the vagina, and exert very gentle downward traction on the pelvic floor muscles about 2 cm inside the introitus, then explain that this is the

TABLE 2.1. Pelvic Floor Assessment Grading

0 = Nil
1 = Muscle on stretch—flicker
2 = Weak squeeze with 2-second hold
3 = Fair squeeze and 5-second hold with lift
4 = Goodsqueeze and 7-second hold and lift, repeats × 5
5 = Strong squeeze and 10-second hold with lift, repeats × 10

muscle we want to contract. We find it helpful to ask the patient to pretend that she is in a public place (church or movie theater) and feels wind building up in the rectum, and to tighten the muscles around the rectum to stop the wind escaping. Most patients have a rough idea of what you are talking about and give a small contraction. You then encourage them by explaining that this is the correct muscle, and explain that now you are going to ask them to contract the muscle as hard as possible and count the number of seconds that they can hold on. The strength of the contraction and the duration are recorded as the modified Oxford Score (Table 2.1).

Once you have assessed the strength and duration of the pelvic floor contraction, you can start the patient on a pelvic floor muscle training program (see Chapter 6).

DO ALL UROGYNECOLOGY PATIENTS NEED A RECTAL EXAMINATION?

Patients with a fairly simple history of stress and/or urge incontinence do not really require a rectal examination, which is uncomfortable and embarrassing. If you suspect neurological disease (which can affect anal function), or the patient has anal incontinence, a rectal exam to assess the tone and quality of the external anal sphincter is often useful. Fecal impaction is often palpable as hard lumps of feces impinging on the posterior wall of the vagina during the assessment of the pelvic floor muscles.

SCREENING NEUROLOGICAL EXAMINATION

If a patient has a history of trauma to the lumbosacral region, or neurological symptoms that have not been investigated, a basic neurological exam is important. The lumbosacral region is of most interest.

The power of the lower limbs, the deep tendon reflexes at the heels, and the sensation of the perineal skin (S4), the skin over the inner lower thigh (S3), or the mid inner thigh (S2) should be checked. Inspect and palpate the lumbosacral spine (sacral dimple may suggest spinal dysraphism; sacral lipoma may be seen). Lightly stroking the skin just beside the anus should provoke a slight contraction of the anus. After explanation, lightly tapping the clitoris should also cause the anus to contract (the bulbocavernosus reflex). After clothing is replaced, observe the patient's gait. If these simple tests are abnormal, a full exam by a neurologist is worthwhile. For a good overview, see Rushton.[1]

Reference
1. Rushton D (1997) Neurological disorders. In: Cardozo L (ed) Urogynaecology, Churchill Livingston, NewYork, pp 481–502.

Chapter 3
How to Manage the Patient After History and Examination

First, Treat Precipitating Factors
The complete management of incontinence and prolapse is not just a surgical exercise! You need to think about the patient's medical problems as they relate to their pelvic floor problem. Collaboration with physicians and other surgeons may be needed. From a medical point of view, referral to a respiratory physician, endocrinologist (for hypothyroid-related obesity, diabetes), dietician, or neurologist may be required. From a surgical point of view, referral to an ENT surgeon, thyroid surgeon, or colorectal surgeon may be needed. The urogynecologist should treat constipation and atrophic vaginal symptoms.

All patients should have a midstream urine cultured to exclude cystitis as a confounding variable/factor that is likely to worsen incontinence (see Chapter 11).

Second, Obtain all Relevant Old Notes
Previous continence surgery needs to be precisely documented, so that you can assess the likelihood of "natural failure" of the procedure, or the risk of post-operative voiding difficulty that may not be symptomatic.

Any previous major abdominal surgery needs to be clarified, especially radical surgery for malignancy, as this may disturb the local innervation, or relays between the sympathetic and parasympathetic nerves in the pelvis, leading to complex incontinence.

Third, Begin a Basic Management Program for Urinary Incontinence
If the condition is mild, this may be curative (see Chapter 5 for definition of mild etc). If the condition is severe or complex, uro-

dynamic tests will be required, but there may be a waiting time for this, hence the need to start basic continence therapy.

- If mild stress incontinence and good PFM strength, give home PFM training program (Chapter 6).
- If mild stress incontinence but weak PFM strength, refer to physiotherapist for electrostimulation; see patients after 12 weeks therapy, book urodynamics then if no cure.
- If severe primary stress incontinence (wants surgery) book urodynamic testing; discuss Tension-Free Vaginal Tape briefly.
- If mild urge incontinence (or just OAB syndrome, not wet) start bladder training program (Chapter 7) and consider referral to nurse continence advisor for detailed training.
- If severe urge incontinence and if long wait for urodynamics tests, give therapeutic trial of anticholinergic drugs, with bladder training (patient to stop drugs one week before test).

Fourth, If Anal Incontinence Is Present
Consider referral to appropriate physiotherapist if mild (Chapter 8). If severe, consider referral to colorectal surgeon for anorectal testing.

Fifth, If Prolapse Symptoms Are Present
If mild symptoms and on examination, consider referral to physiotherapist. Treatment of precipitating factors can make cure much more likely. If there is a moderate or severe prolapse, assess suitability for surgery and patient's wishes (see Chapter 10). Discuss vaginal ring pessary or surgery as indicated. Ensure postmenopausal women are given topical estrogens prior to ring or surgery.

If Associated Recurrent Bacterial Cystitis (Urinary Tract Infection, UTI) Is Present
Obtain old MSU results where possible to check for proven UTI. Order renal ultrasound and post-void residual measurement (Chapter 11). Consider booking uroflowmetry for next visit, if urodynamic tests not needed.

If Suprapubic Pain, with Severe Frequency, Urgency, and Nocturia Is Present
Consider diagnosis of interstitial cystitis (Chapter 12). Make sure the urine is sterile. Check that the frequency volume chart documents the severity of symptoms. Consider booking a cystoscopy with refill examination +/– biopsy.

A FEW WORDS ABOUT EXPLAINING THE SITUATION TO THE PATIENT

Urinary Incontinence

Most patients have little idea that there are different kinds of leakage. We find it helpful to give out a short booklet explaining this at the end of the first visit, which describes the symptoms, underlying causes, and treatments of stress, urge, and overflow incontinence. It is very helpful to explain that, using a step-by-step approach, most urinary incontinence is largely curable, but that it will not happen overnight. You need to be very sympathetic during this explanation, emphasizing how common the problem is (10% of all women under age 65, 25% of women over age 65, and 30% of women who have recently delivered a baby), so that the patient realizes she is not alone in her problem.

Anal Incontinence

Almost all patients with this problem are deeply embarrassed. Again, it is helpful to explain that there are different causes for this condition; treatment needs to be according to the cause and thus investigation is very helpful. Although cure is not as uniformly guaranteed, major improvement is generally likely to occur.

Prolapse

Many patients have little idea of their anatomy, which walls/organs may be involved in prolapse, and that severity of each one does vary. We find it extremely helpful to draw a diagram for the patient, illustrating her particular problem, and showing her degree of severity. If surgery is indicated/desired, the relevant procedures should also be sketched simply on the diagram (see Chapter 10).

Explanations of UTI and IC are given in Chapters 11 and 12.

Chapter 4

How to Conduct Urodynamic Studies: Essentials of a Good Urodynamic Report

WHO NEEDS URODYNAMIC TESTING?

Urodynamic testing is an invasive procedure. At the minimum a urethral catheter and a rectal balloon must be inserted. The risk of iatrogenic bacterial cystitis is about 2%. Recent studies have suggested that urodynamic testing is not cost effective in all patients with urinary leakage, because it does not always affect management.

On the other hand, it is fair to say that performing incontinence surgery without having a urodynamic diagnosis of stress incontinence, excluding detrusor overactivity, and checking for voiding difficulty, is not good medical practice at all. Several studies have shown that simply having a main complaint of stress incontinence does not equate to the patient having urodynamic stress incontinence (USI).

As is explained further in Chapter 9 (surgery for USI), the fact that a cough can provoke a detrusor contraction was a major stimulus for the establishment of urogynecology as a subspecialty. Gynecologists realized that simply operating on patients who leak when they cough is fraught with difficulty.

So one needs to take a stance midway between "urodynamics for everyone" (not warranted because of the invasiveness of the procedure) and urodynamics only for those who are surgical candidates. In practice the real problem is that so many patients have mixed symptoms. Urodynamic results do help to dissect out the relative severity of the different components in patients with mixed incontinence, and thus guide you as to the main thrust of treatment. This is described in the case history at the end of this chapter.

In general, urodynamics are very worthwhile in the following cases (in descending order).

■ Patients with *failed continence surgery* need detailed urodynamic studies.

■ Patients with symptoms or a past history of *voiding difficulty* (previous prolonged catheter or self-catheterization post-op or post-partum) need voiding cystometry.

■ Patients with *mixed symptoms and cystocele* who are considering surgery should have detailed urodynamics, possibly with ring pessary in situ (see "Occult" Stress Incontinence).

■ Patients with *mixed stress and urge leak* need cystometry at least, to determine the relative severity of the two problems.

■ Patients with *pure stress incontinence symptoms who have failed physiotherapy* should have cystometry with some form of imaging, to check whether there is undiagnosed detrusor overactivity or incomplete emptying.

■ Patients with *pure urge symptoms who have failed bladder training and anticholinergic therapy* should also have cystometry with imaging, to look for an undiagnosed stress incontinence component or incomplete emptying (the latter may be worsened by the anticholinergic drugs).

DIFFERENT FORMS OF URODYNAMIC STUDIES

The term "urodynamics" is a general phrase, used to describe a group of tests that assess the filling and voiding phase of the micturition reflex, to determine specific abnormalities.

Some of these tests are not "physiological". For example, inserting catheters into the urethra and a pressure balloon into the rectum, then expecting the patient to fill and empty as she normally does, may not give a "true" picture of that woman's micturition cycle. Nevertheless, the tests have been standardized over the years, in accordance with the Standardization Committee of the International Continence Society (ICS), and are performed in a similar fashion across the world. Therefore abnormalities are interpreted in a standard way, and have a common meaning in clinical practice.

The tests that are generally used include the following.

Uroflowmetry: Measuring the patient's flow rate when voiding in private, onto a commode that is connected to a collecting device that measures the rate of fall of urine upon the device.

Simple cystometry: Inserting a single catheter into the bladder that measures pressure, with no correction for abdominal pressure, during a filling cycle. Not widely used in the Western world.

Twin channel subtracted cystometry: Inserting a pressure recording line into the bladder, as well as a filling catheter, along with an abdominal pressure recording line (rectal balloon), that records a filling cycle. The abdominal pressure is subtracted from the bladder pressure to give the detrusor pressure (see Figure 4.1 and later figures).

Voiding cystometry: The same as twin channel cystometry above, but the patient is asked to void into a uroflow commode while the pressure lines are in situ, so that the contractility of the detrusor muscle during the voiding phase is measured.

Videourodynamics: The same as voiding cystometry above, but radio-opaque X-ray contrast dye is used to fill the bladder. The test is done in the X-ray department, and the bladder/urethra is filmed during cough and other provocation. In males, filming is continued during the voiding phase, but 60% of women are not able to void in these public conditions. Post-void films are taken to check residual.

Voiding cystometry with ultrasound: The same as voiding cystometry, but ultrasound imaging is undertaken during cough and other provocation, and post-void image is taken.

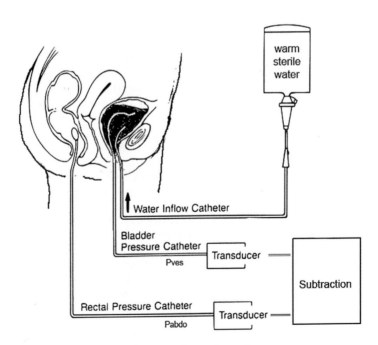

FIGURE 4.1. Schematic diagram of twin channel cystometry.

Urethral pressure profile: Tests the function of the external urethral sphincter, performed in selected cases. Similar information is available from *leak point pressure* testing.

The frequency volume chart and the pad test are also part of
urodynamic assessment, but these are discussed in Chapter 5
(Outcome Measures).

PRACTICAL ADVICE ABOUT HOW TO PERFORM URODYNAMIC STUDIES

This section gives practical advice for a registrar or resident/
house officer who is newly attached to a urogynecology department. For information about the medical physics of the tests,
books by Abrams[1] or Cardozo and Staskin[5] are recommended.

Calibration of the Equipment

In essence, one must check that the equipment is correctly func-
tioning and measures what it is supposed to measure.

Calibration of the urine flow machine involves pouring a
known quantity of fluid into the uroflow equipment at a reason-
ably slow rate, and then checking that the volume poured in
equals the volume measured, and that the computer calculated
the flow rate correctly.

Calibration of the cystometry equipment involves checking
that a column of fluid 100 cm high yields a pressure reading of
100 cm H_2O water pressure, then zeroing the transducers to
atmospheric pressure (room air) so that zero pressure gives a
zero reading. For detailed discussion, see suggested further
reading.

General Clinical Guidelines

When a patient presents for urodynamics studies, you need to
"troubleshoot" to make sure that the test can be correctly performed on the day.

If she has symptoms of acute urinary tract infection (dysuria,
foul-smelling urine, excessive frequency, strangury, or hematuria), then the test should be abandoned, a midstream urine
culture taken, and antibiotics prescribed. This is because instru-
mentation of the lower urinary tract in the presence of infection
can cause septicemia.

In many Units, there is a substantial delay between the first
visit date and the date of the urodynamic test. In these cases,
you should review the patient's status quickly before starting the
test.

If the patient was given a therapeutic trial of anticholinergic therapy at the first visit, but was not given clear instructions to stop them 1–3 weeks before the test (and is still taking them), then cystometry may not diagnose detrusor overactivity.

If the patient had mild symptoms and has been attending a physiotherapist or nurse continence advisor in the meantime, she may be cured of her incontinence and no longer need the test.

Explaining the Test to the Patient

This is best done by the urodynamics nurse, who must form a trusting relationship with the patient. In our Unit, that same nurse may have been involved in taking her initial history, or will often be involved in following up the patient's response to treatment subsequently.

Urodynamic testing does involve some minor discomfort with passage of urethral and rectal catheters, but if performed in a dignified and sympathetic manner, most patients say that it was just slightly uncomfortable. In a teaching unit, only one medical student should "watch" the procedure. Actually we ask the student to position the lamp, type in data on the computer, help the patient off the couch, so they do not "watch" the patient but are actively involved. Patients do not like to feel like a goldfish in a bowl, especially when they are being asked to leak.

Before starting to fill, the nurse or doctor also explains the concepts of First Desire to Void, Strong Desire to Void, and Maximum Cystometric Capacity (see below). It is important for patients to know we will stop filling if they have too much discomfort.

UROFLOWMETRY

Ideally, the patient should come to the urodynamics test with a comfortably full bladder, then pass urine in a private uroflowmetry cubicle. Because many patients empty their bladder just before seeing a doctor, this is not always possible (no matter what letter you send beforehand).

A normal urine flow rate (shown in Figure 4.2) looks like a bell-shaped tracing. The maximum flow rate should be at least 15 ml/sec, but this cannot be judged unless the voided volume is at least 150 to 200 ml. This is because flow rate depends on the volume in the bladder. For example, if you drink several pints of beer, you will pass urine rapidly. If you only drink the occasional small cup of tea, your flow rate will trickle out.

Normal values for flow rate in relation to volume voided have been derived from a study of several hundred normal women

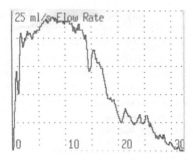

FIGURE 4.2. Normal uroflow curve. Maximum flow rate 23 ml/sec, average 14 ml/sec, voided volume 410 mls, Flow time 31 sec.

(Haylen et al;[6] see Figure 4.3). These "Nomograms" allow you to determine what centile of the population a patient's flow rate represents. Flow rates below the tenth centile are considered abnormal.

Other parameters that are measured include the total duration of flow time to empty the bladder, and the average flow rate (that is the volume voided divided by the flow time).

Typical abnormalities of flow rate in women include intermittent prolonged flow rate with evidence of abdominal straining, suggestive of outflow obstruction. This most commonly

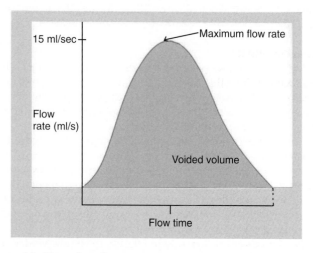

FIGURE 4.3. Normal uroflow parameters.

occurs after surgery for stress incontinence that has over-compensated the urethral support. It is also seen in women with a cystourethrocele, in which the urethra may be kinked during voiding.

The other common abnormality in elderly women is an underactive detrusor; see Figure 4.4. The peak flow rate is poor, the average flow rate is poor, but there is no evidence of abdominal straining. The detrusor contraction is intrinsically weak, but this needs to be proven by voiding cystometry.

Less common voiding abnormalities are described in the section on voiding cystometry (detrusor hyperactivity with impaired contractility, DHIC, seen in the elderly with mild neurological dysfunction, and detrusor sphincter dyssynergia, seen only in neuropathic disease such as multiple sclerosis).

After uroflowmentry, residual urine volume is measured either by catheterization, if the patient is about to undergo cystometry, or by ultrasound. A simple "bladder scan" (Bard) may be used, which automatically calculates the residual volume. Alternatively, standard trans-abdominal or trans-vaginal ultrasound is used to measure the residual volume, and formulae that calculate the volume of a sphere are then used by the clinician to calculate the residual amount (eg width × depth × height × 0.7).

Performance of Cystometry

To pass the bladder catheters, the urethra is cleansed with sterile saline, a sterile drape is placed around the urethra, lignocaine gel is applied to the urethra, then the filling line and the pressure recording line (similar to a Central Venous Pressure manometry line) are inserted into the urethra. Usually, the manometry line is inserted into the distal catheter hole, so the patient only feels one line going into the urethra, then the manometry line is disconnected from the filling line by pulling it backwards slightly once it is in the bladder. The vesical pressure line is then attached to the domed transducer unit, which feeds into the software of the urodynamic equipment. See Figure 4.5.

Some Units employ a catheter that has a micro-tip pressure transducer embedded into the distal end, so that an external transducer is not needed, and the slight artifactual delay encountered in the fluid-filled system is avoided. Such micro-tip transducer catheters are quite costly (1500 to 1800 Euros per catheter) and are quite delicate, so they may last roughly six months to two years of normal use. The fluid-filled pressure recording lines are single-use items, costing a few Euros per set. Each Unit

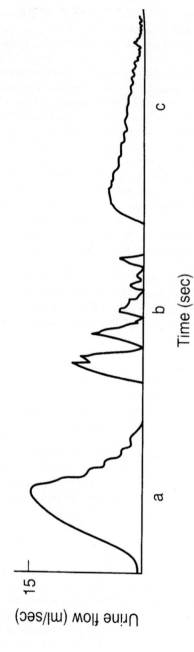

FIGURE 4.4. (A) Normal. (B) Abdominal straining. (C) Underactive detrusor. (Reprinted with permission from Prolapse and urinary incontinence. In: Leader LR et al (1996) Handbook of obstetrics and gynaecology, 4th edn. Copyright Chapman & Hall 1996 p. 406; Reproduced by permissions of Edward Arnold.)

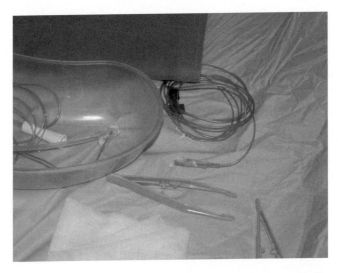

FIGURE 4.5. Bladder filling line, vesical pressure line, and rectal balloon.

makes its own decision about which catheter type to use, generally on the basis of cost.

Passing the Rectal Catheter

The rectal balloon is attached to the abdominal pressure recording line (either pre-packaged by the manufacturer, or a glove finger stall is tied on with suture, to save costs). The balloon is coated in sterile lubricant, then placed into the rectum. Do not push your finger into the patient's rectum; this is unpleasant and unnecessary. Just gently insert the balloon about 3 cm into the rectal ampulla. A vaginal balloon may also be used to record intra-vaginal pressure which is equivalent, but this is usually not successful in parous women as the balloon slips out in the erect position.

TWIN CHANNEL CYSTOMETRY

After connecting the bladder pressure recording line and the abdominal pressure recording line to the transducer dome, insert fluid into the line to exclude air bubbles, then zero the recording pressure using the software of the urodynamic program. The software program will subtract the abdominal pressure (Pabdo) from the vesical pressure (Pves) to yield the true detrusor pressure (Pdet).

The bladder is then filled with warm sterile water. Medium filling rate (10–100 ml) is advised in nonneuropathic patients. Generally a rate of 50–75 ml is used, via a peristaltic pump to prevent backflow into the bladder during a rise in detrusor pressure. The following parameters are important in a full urodynamic report.

- Results of free uroflowmetry if available.
- *Initial residual* urine volume (after the patient has performed free uroflowmetry).
  —Normal residual = less than 50 ml.
- Whether *pain or resistance* to catheterization is noted (may suggest urethral stenosis).
- The *first desire to void*, when patient first notes that she would look for a toilet.
  —Normal FDV = 150–200 ml.
- *Normal desire*, when patient would normally stop work and go to toilet.
  —Normal desire usually = 350–400 ml.
- *Maximum cystometric capacity*, when patient would not tolerate any more fluid. Although the patient should not be pushed to the point of bladder pain, we use the example that if she were driving in the country she would get out of her car and go behind the bushes to void.
  —Normal MCC = 450–500 ml.
- The filling line is then removed (because it has a diameter sufficient to obstruct the outflow of urine during the next steps).
- A supine cough is performed, while the urethra is visually inspected to look for a *stress leak*. Reassure the patient that there is only sterile water in the bladder, and that all linen is discarded after each test regardless, so she will not spoil the linen. At this point, a *cough-provoked detrusor contraction* may be seen.
- *Supine tapwater provocation* is performed, while asking if urgency is increased by the sound of running water (and rise in detrusor pressure is checked for).
- The patient then stands erect.
- The transducer levels are readjusted so that they remain at the level of the symphysis pubis (e.g. raise them for a tall patient).
- *Erect tapwater* stimulus is performed (as for supine).
- *Erect cough* is performed, with the legs widely apart. Reassure the patient that if any fluid escapes, it is only sterile water, there is no urine in the bladder, and this is an important part of the test.

■ The patient then sits down on the uroflow commode, the transducers are lowered so they remain at the symphysis pubis, and *voiding cystometry* commences.

URODYNAMIC DIAGNOSES AVAILABLE FROM THE FILLING PHASE

The diagnoses that may be made during the filling phase (Abrams et al[2]) are as follows.

Urodynamic stress incontinence (USI) is the involuntary leakage of fluid during increased abdominal pressure, in the absence of a detrusor contraction (Figure 4.6).

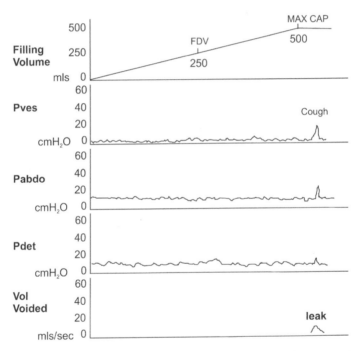

FIGURE 4.6. Urodynamic stress incontinence, with a normal FDV, SDV, and MCC, no detrusor contractions (Pves and Pdet remain flat) but obvious leak of fluid with cough.

Detrusor overactivity is a urodynamic observation characterizd by involuntary detrusor contractions during the filling phase which may be spontaneous or provoked. The most common picture is that of systolic detrusor pressure waves, seen during the filling phase (Figure 4.7). The same picture is seen when the sound of running tapwater provokes a detrusor contraction.

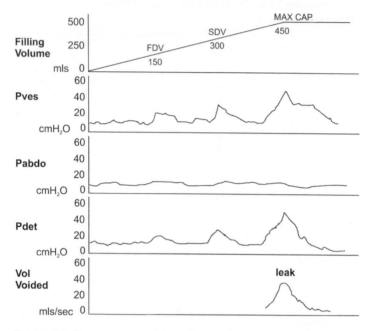

FIGURE 4.7. Detrusor overactivity with systolic waves of detrusor contractions, seen at FDV and at MCC. Stress leak does not occur.

A less well understood phenomenon is detrusor overactivity (Figure 4.8) seen as a gradual linear rise in bladder pressure, that persists after filling stops, in association with urgency. This is often termed *"low compliance DO"*.

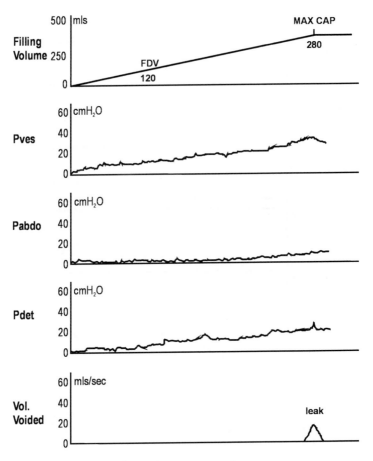

FIGURE 4.8. Low compliance detrusor overactivity.

Finally, two less common but important variants of systolic overactivity are cough-provoked DO and erect-provoked DO. Cough-provoked DO is usually quite clearly seen on the tracing (Figure 4.9).

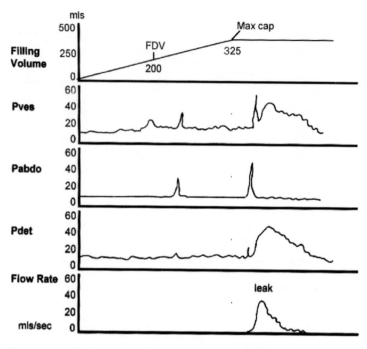

FIGURE 4.9. Cough-provoked detrusor overactivity.

But erect provoked DO often needs careful scrutiny to exclude arti-
fact. A common problem is that the abdominal pressure transducer is not readjusted when the patient stands up (it is not
re-positioned to the level of the pubic symphysis). If a short
patient stands up from the table, her pubic bone may drop to
well below its original site when she was lying on the couch;
Pabdo then becomes negative. Because Pves minus Pabdo
equals Pdet, if you subtract a falsely negative Pabdo, you will
get a falsely positive Pdet when the patient stands (see Figure
4.18 given as part of the case history at end of this chapter).

What Is "Sensory Urgency"?

For many years, patients who suffered from frequency, urgency,
and nocturia, in whom urodynamic testing revealed a stable
bladder, but a very early First Desire to Void (less than 100–
150 ml) and a small Maximum Cystometric Capacity (less than 400
ml) were diagnosed as having sensory urgency (Jarvis[9]). These
patients often found bladder filling unduly painful. More recently,

the International Continence Society has moved towards regarding such patients as being on the mild end of the spectrum of "Painful Bladder Syndrome". The severe end of the spectrum of such cases is frank interstitial cystitis.

Another problem arises in that repeat twin channel cystometry (and ambulatory cystometry, a research tool) reveals detrusor overactivity in at least one third of cases of "sensory urgency."

The management of patients with a small capacity stable bladder is therefore usually empirical. One starts out treating as for detrusor overactivity, because they do meet the clinical criteria for the symptom complex of overactive bladder. If the patient doesn't respond, then cystoscopy to look for features of interstitial cystitis is reasonable. This area is controversial.

Features of the Atonic Bladder During the Filling Phase

Patients with a very late FDV (more than 400–500 ml) and a very large MCC (more than 650–750 ml) have characteristics of an atonic bladder, but this condition should not really be diagnosed until voiding cystometry has been performed, to prove that the detrusor is underactive.

Before going on to describe voiding cystometry, a summary of *videourodynamic testing* and twin channel cystometry with *ultrasound imaging* is given.

VIDEOURODYNAMICS

Videourodynamic Testing

This involves installation of a radio-opaque dye (eg Hypaque) dissolved in warm water, while screening intermittently using a fluoroscopy unit with image intensifier in the radiology department. A fluoroscopy table that rises to the erect position is needed, with a platform on the bottom of the table, so that the erect patient can turn to the side for filming of the lateral view of the bladder neck and urethra (see Figure 4.10). This study is termed *videocystourethrography (VCU)* where a videotape can be made of the screening images that most software packages can superimpose upon the cystometry tracing, and store for later review.

Because VCU involves exposure to X-ray, and installation of iodine-containing medium which patients may be allergic to, not to mention the costs of using the fluoroscopy unit, it is only needed in selected cases.

VCU was the initial "gold-standard" urodynamic test, and is still important for male patients in whom prostatic outflow obstruction needs to be delineated from simple detrusor over-

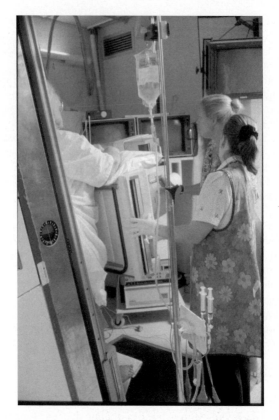

FIGURE 4.10. Patient in erect position during screening on video-cystourethrography.

activity. In men, the voiding phase is always screened. Also, in men with neurological disease, VCU allows clearer definition of any contribution from prostatitic outflow obstruction. Finally, VCU allows detection of vesico-ureteric reflux which may threaten the upper urinary tract.

In the female, studies have shown that about 60% of women cannot void in the upright position on a screening table with a collecting funnel between their legs.

During a cough, the bladder neck may be slightly open, forming the shape of a bird's beak, with fluid entering the proximal urethra (called "beaking"; see Figure 4.11). In more severe cases, the urethra may open widely in the shape of a funnel during cough (called "funneling"). In the worst-case scenario, as soon as the patient stands, the bladder funnels open widely and

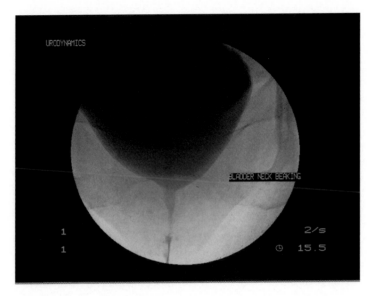

FIGURE 4.11. "Beaking" on VCU.

fluid pours out onto the floor. These findings have been classified using various grading systems (Herschorn[7]).

VCU is very helpful in women with failed previous continence surgery. In the anteroposterior view, typical features of previous colposuspension or sling can be seen, with slightly "dog-ears"-shaped indentation just lateral to the bladder neck. Sometimes although these lateral indentations are partly evident, the urethrovesical junction may still be hypermobile on the lateral view, suggesting that the sutures are no longer effective.

The patient in Figure 4.11 had undergone macroplastique injections to the midurethra, which explains the slightly asymmetrical picture of the "beak."

In other cases, the sutures are very evident; the bladder neck does not open appreciably, but fluid still leaks out. This is typically suggestive of *intrinsic sphincteric deficiency*; ie the urethral musculature is intrinsically weak. Many clinicians would seek to quantify this by performing an Abdominal Leak Point Pressure or a Urethral Pressure Profile (see below).

Value of VCU in Cystocele

In patients symptomatic of cystocele (often worse at the end of the day, not when you examine them in the morning clinic), a cystocele may be very evident in the erect position with a full bladder, that was not clearly seen when examined in the supine

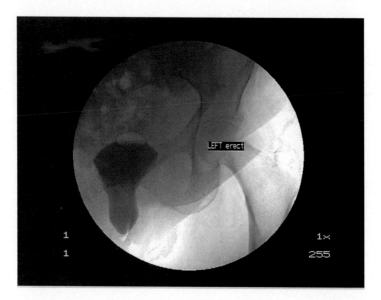

FIGURE 4.12. Urine trapping in a dependant cystocele after voiding.

position. At the end of the voiding phase, you may also see urine trapping in the cystocele (when screening in the erect position to check post-void residual; see Figure 4.12).

"OCCULT" STRESS INCONTINENCE

One problem in urogynecology is that a patient with cystocele but no appreciable incontinence may begin leaking <u>after</u> an anterior repair. This is because the cystocele may involve the upper portion of the urethra, so when the cystocele descends during cough, the urethra is kinked off, masking the incipient incontinence. It is very disturbing when the patient comes to the postoperative visit complaining of stress incontinence for the first time. This is known as "occult" stress incontinence. The likelihood of this occurring ranges from 7–28%, depending upon the publication (for review, see Adekanmi et al[3]).

Such patients may have to replace their cystocele manually before they can have a good stream of urine. If they don't digitate the cystocele, they can have initial hesitancy, need to strain to start, and have terminal dribble. In such cases, it is worthwhile to conduct VCU (or twin channel cystometry) with a ring pessary in situ, as this is likely to unmask the occult incontinence. This allows one to incorporate a specific procedure for incontinence into the repair operation (for discussion see Karram[11]).

ULTRASOUND

Because of the costs and X-ray exposure involved with VCU, ultrasound imaging has become popular as part of urodynamic testing.

Initially, ultrasound imaging of the pelvis used trans-abdominal scanning which gave poor definition of the bladder neck. The next step was to use trans-vaginal scanning, which allowed better definition of the bladder neck but could not be performed during a stress provocation test (because the vaginal probe interfered with urethral leakage). In the last decade, trans-perineal scanning has allowed good visualization of the bladder neck. Using this technique, one can assess the following.

- Hypermobility of the bladder neck region
- Fluid in the proximal urethra
- Beaking and funneling of the urethra

The main difficulties are that

- Ultrasound scanning is not easy to perform in the erect position, and
- Trans-perineal scanning does not easily yield a lateral view that is helpful in previous failed continence surgery.

Therefore trans-perineal scanning occupies an intermediate position in terms of accurate anatomical assessment of complex incontinence (somewhere between simple "eyeballing" of leakage on twin channel cystometry, and full radiological imaging with VCU).

VOIDING CYSTOMETRY

During voiding cystometry, the patient sits on the uroflow commode with the pressure transducers in situ. All staff leave the room while she voids in private (Figure 4.13). The maximum and average flow rates (Q Max and Q Ave) are measured, as in a free uroflow, but the maximum detrusor pressure at the point of maximum flow (Pdet at Q Max) is also measured. The findings may be as follows.

- In outflow obstruction, Q Max and Q Ave are low, but the detrusor pressure is high (the detrusor is trying to overcome the obstruction, so Pdet at Q Max is high, called "high pressure, low flow").
- Also in outflow obstruction, abdominal straining may be seen on Pabdo channel.
- In an underactive detrusor, the Q Max and Q Ave are low, but the detrusor pressure at Q Max is also low (called "low pressure, low flow"), which is a feature of the atonic bladder.

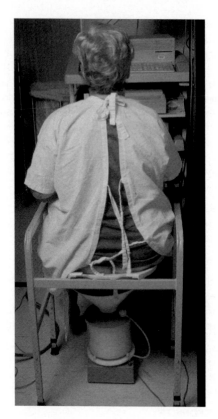

FIGURE 4.13. Voiding cystometry.

Diagnoses Made After Voiding Cystometry

Outflow Obstruction

In women the most common cause of obstruction is previous continence surgery or prolapse kinking the urethra (see Figure 4.14). The high detrusor pressure with the low flow rate is typical. If sufficient voiding efficiency can be generated (often with abdominal straining, giving an intermittent pattern) then the residual may be minimal.

Atonic Bladder

As mentioned, some features of bladder atony (large volume at FDV and MCC) are seen during filling, but during voiding, the most important feature emerges, of low detrusor pressure with low flow rate. Generally there is a substantial residual. In women,

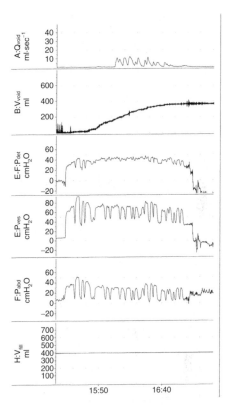

FIGURE 4.14. Obstructed voiding pattern on voiding cystometry. Note detrusor contracting vigorously, then abdominal straining added, to achieve bladder emptying. Although flow was intermittent and prolonged, the residual was 40 ml (Qvoid = flowrate, ml/sec).

this may be seen with diabetic autonomic neuropathy, or it may be a marker of a neurological lesion at the level of the sacral cord.

Detrusor Hyperactivity with Impaired Contractility (DHIC)

This is another cause of an underactive detrusor in elderly women. During the filling phase, there may be mild detrusor overactivity (see Figure 4.15). During voiding, there is an initial burst of detrusor activity at the start of flow (detrusor hyperactivity), but it is not sustained through the whole flow (impaired contractility). This condition is thought to be due to atherosclerotic changes of the blood vessels supplying the spinal cord, so that there is relative impairment of the coordination of the micturition reflex (Resnick and Yalla[13]).

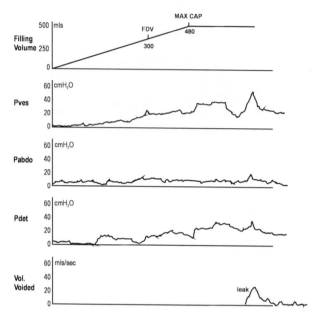

FIGURE 4.15. Detrusor hyperactivity with impaired contractility. Note detrusor overactivity during filling phase, but poorly sustained contractility during voiding. Q Max 8 ml/sec, Q Ave 3.5 ml/sec, and residual volume was 120 ml.

Detrusor Sphincter Dyssynergia (DSD)

In women with multiple sclerosis or spinal cord injury, you may see severe detrusor overactivity during the filling phase, then during voiding, very high detrusor pressures, and an intermittent flow rate without abdominal straining, due to intermittent spasm of the urethra. It is due to poor coordination of the spinal relays of the impulses that signal the command to void. These should evoke synchronous relaxation of the urethra with contraction of the detrusor, but in DSD the synchrony is impaired due to spinal cord pathology (for review see Jung and Chancellor[10] 2001).

SPECIAL URODYNAMIC TESTS

Urethral Pressure Profilometry

With about 200 ml fluid in the bladder, a double lumen fluid-filled manometry catheter, or a flexible micro-tipped pressure recording catheter with one transducer mounted at the end and one 6 cm along, is withdrawn from the bladder into the urethra. A mechanical puller device is used so that withdrawal occurs at about 5–10 cm/min. First a *resting urethral pressure profile (UPP)* is made, to record the rise in pressure as the catheter at the 6 cm position passes through the urethral sphincter area. See Figure 4.16. The urethral closure pressure equals urethral pressure

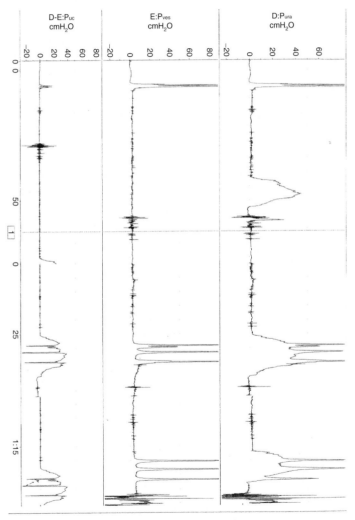

* ☐ 1 1:01 maximun urethral closing pressure =40

FIGURE 4.16. Urethral pressure profile test in stress incontinence.

(Pura) minus the bladder pressure (Pves). In a continent woman, Pura exceeds Pves. In most continent women the urethral closure pressure is greater than 60 cm H_2O pressure (although the UPP has been criticized because there is no absolute cut-off between continence and incontinence for this test). A resting closure pressure of less than 20 cm H_2O is considered very low, and is one indicator of *intrinsic sphincteric deficiency (ISD)*.

Next the catheter is re-inserted into the bladder and withdrawn through the urethra while the patient gives a series of short hard coughs (a *"stress UPP"*). Even while coughing, Pura should exceed Pves. In the incontinent woman, the Pves repeatedly exceeds the Pura during the cough, yielding a "negative stress profile."

Abdominal or Valsalva Leak Point Pressure Test

At a volume of 200–250 ml, with a simple manometry line in the bladder (as for cystometry set-up), the patient is asked to give a series of progressively harder coughs or Valsalva maneuvers. The intravesical pressure required to produce leakage from the external meatus (in the absence of a detrusor contraction) is called the Leak Point Pressure (LPP). An LPP of less than 60 cm is thought to indicate *intrinsic sphincteric deficiency:* 60–100 cm H_2O is equivocal, and a pressure of more than 100 cm is often taken to indicate that the leak is due to urethral hypermobility. The test is controversial because test–retest reliability has been difficult to document, and correlation with other measures of incontinence severity is not high.

Triple Lumen (Trantner) Catheter Test for Urethral Diverticulum

This test is performed using radiological screening. A triple lumen catheter with two balloons, and one lumen for radio-opaque dye that fills the urethra, is used (see Figure 4.17). A smaller balloon is filled with 5–8 ml water and compressed gently against the internal urethral meatus. A larger balloon is filled with 20 ml of water and compressed against the external urethral meatus, so that fluid cannot escape the urethra except under considerable pressure. Radio-opaque dye is injected into the urethra. If a urethral diverticulum exists, with a patent lumen from the diverticulum into the urethra, the dye will run into the diverticulum. During screening with a rotating C-arm, the location of the diverticulum can be pinpointed.

Although excluding the diagnosis of urethral diverticulum is an important part of urogynecology investigation, the condition is not commonly encountered (about 3% of women with lower urinary tract symptoms). Therefore it is not further discussed in

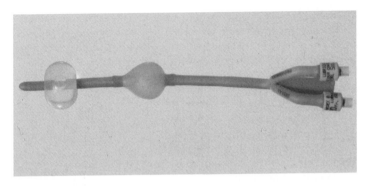

FIGURE 4.17. Triple lumen Trantner Catheter.

this "practical" text (but see Nichols and Randall[12] or Cardozo[4] for full review).

Note Regarding Diagnostic Tests for Vesicovaginal Fistulae

Because vesicovaginal fistulae are not common in the Western world, details of diagnosis and management are outside the scope of this text. For full review, see Hilton.[8]

EXAMPLE OF REPORT

Case History, with Example of a Full Urodynamic Report, Illustrating Contribution of Urodynamic Studies to Management

Mrs. Brown is a 47-year-old para 2 + 0 lady. Ten years ago, after her second delivery (Kiellands forceps) she noted leakage with standing up from the sitting position, with mixed stress and urge incontinence. She had twin channel cystometry elsewhere; results are lost. Afterwards, she was given six weeks of Ditropan 5 mg TDS, which she did not tolerate because of dry mouth. Pelvic floor physiotherapy was not performed. She told the doctor she did not want any more tablets but would like an operation. She underwent a colposuspension, and went home with a suprapubic catheter for ten days.

She was dry for about two years, but did notice persistent daytime urge with nocturia. Since then, she has had gradually increasing leakage when arising from a sitting position. She often has to go back to the toilet to revoid.

On examination, with bladder partly full, stress leak is not seen. The anterior vaginal wall is not hypermobile. The retropubic area is rather fixed to the back of the pubic bone, more so on the left than the right. She had a weak 2 sec pelvic floor contraction.

Summary: This patient may have failed continence surgery with recurrent stress leak, or she may have an overactive bladder, or she may have both. Obstruction is also a possibility to explain her need to revoid. Clearly, careful urodynamics are essential.

Urodynamic Result

Initial Residual: 90 ml.

> —First desire to void = 190 ml.
> —Strong desire to void = 230 ml.
> —Maximum capacity = 380 ml.

During filling phase, systolic detrusor contractions were seen, Max P det of 21 cm.

Supine tapwater = increase in Pdet to 28 cm H_2O.

Supine cough = no stress leak.

Erect provocation = increased detrusor pressure to Pdet 35 cm H_2O with leak.

During multiple erect coughs, the patient leaked a small amount of fluid; on screening, asymmetrical beaking of the bladder neck was seen, with fluid leak.

In lateral view, the bladder neck did not descend.

Voiding cystometry

> —Q Max 25 ml/sec; Q Ave 9 ml/sec.
> —Flow rate was intermittent and prolonged, with abdominal straining.
> —Pdet at Q Max was 45 cm H_2O; Final residual was 110 ml.

See Figure 4.18.

Comments

Mrs. Brown has a reduced bladder capacity (380 ml), with detrusor contractions provoked by filling, supine tapwater, and erect provocation. She does have some stress incontinence with an asymmetrical appearance of the urethra, in keeping with findings on examining the retropubic vagina. Her maximum flow rate is fine, but her average flow rate is poor, with abdominal straining suggesting relative outflow obstruction, in keeping with initial and final residuals of 90 ml/110 ml.

Diagnosis: Marked Detrusor Overactivity (DO) with Mild Degree of Obstruction; Mild Stress Incontinence

Management

Treat the DO with bladder training, including pelvic floor muscle physiotherapy. Teach double emptying techniques. At six weeks,

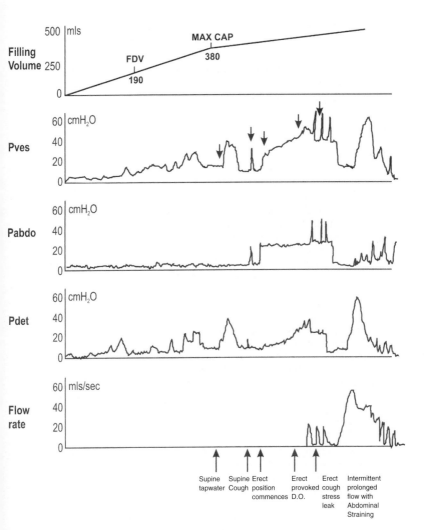

FIGURE 4.18. Urodynamic study of Mrs. Brown.

start anticholinergics, eg tolteridine (less dry mouth), but recheck post-void residual six weeks later. If increased, may need to consider clean intermittent self catheterization. After this therapy, if stress incontinence persists, consider collagen/macroplastique.

Note: If this patient had undergone pelvic floor training initially, with alternative anticholinergic therapy, the current situation may not have arisen.

CONCLUSIONS

Urodynamic testing requires careful attention to detail, both in the selection and counseling of the patient during the test, in performance of the provocation maneuvers, and in analysis of the results, to obtain precise diagnoses of the components of the continence disorder. Unlike an ECG that can be performed by a technician, this test requires a trained clinician in order to yield the maximum information.

References

1. Abrams P (1997) Urodynamics, 2nd edn. Springer, London.
2. Abrams P, Cardozo L, Fall M, Griffiths D, Rosier P, Ulmsten U, et al (2002) The standardisation of terminology of lower urinary tract function: Report from the Standardisation Sub-committee of the International Continence Society. Neurourol Urodyn 21:167–178.
3. Adekanmi OA, Bombieri L, Freeman RM (2001) Occult incontinence: A review. Aust Continence J 7:40–43.
4. Cardozo L (1997) Urethral problems. In: Urogynaecology. Churchill Livingstone, New York, Chapter 24, pp 377–386.
5. Cardozo L, Staskin D, eds (2001) Textbook of female urology and urogynaecology, Martin Dunitz, London, Chapters 17–27, pp 183–312.
6. Haylen BT, Ashby D, Sutherst JR et al (1989) Maximum and average urine flow rates in normal male and female populations—the Liverpool nomograms. Br J Urol 64:30–38.
7. Herschorn S (2001) Videourodynamics. In: Cardozo L and Staskin D (eds), Textbook of Female Urology and Urogynaecology. Martin Dunitz, London, Chapter 24, pp 264–274.
8. Hilton P (2001) Surgical fistulae and obstetric fistulae. In: Cardozo L and Staskin D (eds), Textbook of Female Urology and Urogynaecology. Martin Dunitz, London, Chapters 55, 56, pp 691–720.
9. Jarvis GJ (1982) The management of urinary incontinence due to primary vesical sensory urgency by bladder drill. Br J Urol 54:374–376.
10. Jung SY, Chancellor MB (2001) Neurological disorders. In: Cardozo L and Staskin D (eds), Textbook of female urology and urogynaecology. Martin Dunitz, London, Chapter 65, pp 837–853.
11. Karram MM (1999) What is the optimal anti-incontinence procedure in women with advanced prolapse and "potential" stress incontinence? Int Urogynaecol J 10:1–2.
12. Nichols DH, Randall CL (1996) Urethral diverticulum and fistulae. In: Vaginal surgery, 4th edn. Williams and Wilkins, Baltimore, Chapter 18, pp 422–425.
13. Resnick NM, Yalla SV (1987) Detrusor hyperactivity with impaired contractile function: An urecognized but common cause of incontinence in elderly patients. JAMA 257:3076–3081.

Chapter 5

Outcome Measures Used to Assess Response

INTRODUCTION

In the past, doctors recommended a particular treatment because, in their experience, most patients said that they were "better" after receiving it. In the last two decades, we have realized that this is not good enough. We need objective measures by which we can determine what percentage of patients are "cured" (normal), or at least have greater than 50% reduction in symptoms, after any given treatment.

In this century, outcome measures are going to become even more important, because there is not enough money to fund all health care. Doctors (and administrators) must assess whether one treatment is more effective than another, so that money can be spent on that which is most effective. This is loosely termed "health economics".

In the 1980s, continence clinicians began to realize the importance of outcome measures. It was a time of great creation. Many different outcome measures were created, but not necessarily fully "validated". The process of validation involves the following steps.

- Establish the validity of the test, that it measures what it is supposed to.
  —Includes three subsets; content validity, construct validity, and criterion validity.
- Establish the reliability of the test.
  —For questionnaires, measure internal consistency of different parts of test.
  —For questionnaires and other physical tests, the reproducibility, or test–retest reliability needs to be proven.
- Establish the responsiveness to change of the test, before and after treatment.

This chapter provides a brief overview of outcome measures that have been validated. Most are used in this book to describe the effectiveness of different treatments.

The Standardization Committee of the International Continence Society (ICS) is the main body that has governed terminology and outcome measures in the field of urinary incontinence since 1978.[8] The urodynamic measures described in the previous chapter, and the pelvic floor assessments (Oxford Score and POPQ) described in Chapter Two, are also used as outcome measures. The tests described in this chapter do not require physical examination or invasive procedures.

The World Health Organization has recently acknowledged the global importance of incontinence, by holding a regular International Consultation on Incontinence (ICI) (Abrams et al[1-3]). These publications also consider which treatments are the most effective, as judged by standardized outcome measures. Finally, the Cochrane Collaboration performs meta-analyses of randomized controlled trials in the field of incontinence, which also use the outcome measures described in this text.

The ICS recommends that there should be five main groups, or "domains" of outcome measures.

1. Patient's observations (symptoms)
2. Quantification of symptoms (eg urine loss on diary or pad test)
3. Physician's observations (anatomical and functional)
4. Quality of life measures
5. Socioeconomic evaluations

TESTS THAT MEASURE PATIENT'S SYMPTOMS

The ICIQ-SF was validated under the auspices of the ICI. It records incontinence symptoms and severity, with a simple quality of life question. The final ICIQ comprises three scored items (Figure 5.1, maximum score 21) and an unscored self-diagnostic item.

ICIQ-SF
Confidential

□□ □□ □□
DAY MONTH YEAR
Today's Date

Many people leak urine some of the time. We are trying to find out how many people leak urine, and how much this bothers them. We would be grateful if you could answer the following questions, thinking about how you have been, on average, over the PAST FOUR WEEKS.

1. **Please write in your date of birth:**

□□ □□ □□
DAY MONTH YEAR

2. **Are you:** *(tick one):*   Female □   Male □

3. **How often do you leak urine?** *(Tick one box)*

Never □ 0
about once a week or less often □ 1
two or three times a week □ 2
about once a day □ 3
several times a day □ 4
all the time □ 5

4. **We would like to know how much urine <u>you think</u> leaks.**
How much urine do you <u>usually</u> leak (whether you wear protection or not)?
(Tick one box)

none □ 0
a small amount □ 2
a moderate amount □ 4
a large amount □ 6

5. **Overall, how much does leaking urine interfere with your everyday life?**
Please ring a number between 0 (not at all) and 10 (a great deal)

0   1   2   3   4   5   6   7   8   9   10
not at all   a great deal

ICIQ score: sum scores 3+4+5 □ □

FIGURE 5.1. The ICIQ-SF Questionnaire.

The Wexner Score for Fecal Incontinence

This was originally a 20-point score concerning three types of incontinence with one question for impact upon lifestyle (italic bold in Table 5.1). Later a score for wearing pads, taking constipating medication, or suffering from fecal urgency were added (ordinary typeface in Table 5.1). The Wexner Score has been fully validated[10] and is used worldwide.

TABLE 5.1. Modified Wexner Fecal Incontinence Score

	Never	Rarely	Sometimes	Weekly	Daily
Incontinent solid stool	0	1	2	3	4
Incontinent liquid stool	0	1	2	3	4
Incontinent to gas	0	1	2	3	4
Alters lifestyle	0	1	2	3	4

	No	Yes
Need to wear pad/plug	0	2
Take constipating meds	0	2
Unable to defer 15 min	0	2

TESTS THAT QUANTIFY PATIENTS' SYMPTOMS

Rather than giving the patient a questionnaire about her symptoms, the following tests actually measure symptoms such as stress leak, urge leak, frequency, or nocturia.

BLADDER CHART

The Bladder Chart is a generic term used to indicate several types of records.

- The *micturition chart* only asks patients to record times of voiding and incontinence episodes; only output is considered, roughly.
- The *frequency volume chart (FVC)* also asks patients to record their fluid intake and the volume they void, and when they change pads, usually over three days.
- The *urinary diary* includes the details of the FVC but also includes symptoms and activities at leakage episodes, including urgency, coughing, lifting, and others.

The micturition chart tells nothing about people who drink too much (>3 liters per day) or too little (<1.5 liters per day). Most clinicians use the Frequency Volume Chart (see Figure 5.2). Although the Urinary Diary (Figure 5.2) provides even more detail about the type of leakage, patients often object to the detail required, depending on how many days of charting you require.

The FVC is a useful outcome measure. It tells you:

- The number of leakage episodes per 24 hours (in mild cases, convert to leaks per week by taking an average of the three days).
- The number of voids per day ("frequency").
- The episodes of nocturia.
- Whether patients are fluid restricting for fear of urge leak.

BLADDER CHART – 1 day (24 Hours)

TIME	AMOUNT & TYPE OF FLUID IN	TIME	AMOUNT OF URINE PASSED	COMMENTS Eg leakage, urge, pain, burning etc.
7:30am	—	7:30 am	290 ml	Leaked on way to toilet ++ urge
7:40	150ml black Coffee			
		8:45	75 ml	urge
9:15	250ml coke			
		9:30	160 ml	leaked on way to toilet urge ++
		10:05	75 ml	urge
		10:40	90 ml	urge
11:00	Capuccino 200ml			
		11:20	110 ml	urge
12:30pm	300ml Soup			
		1:15pm	230 ml	leak with laughing
		3:30pm	60ml	leak at photocopier
3:40	75ml espresso			
		4:45pm	50 ml	urge
		6:30pm	85 ml	
7:00	90ml sherry			
		8:05pm	100	leak with washing dishes
		11:30pm	120	woken from sleep.
		02:30	65	

FIGURE 5.2. A urinary diary from a patient with urge incontinence. Patient drinks little (1.065 l/day), has marked frequency (11 voids/day), nocturia × 2, and a small bladder capacity (average of 12 voids = 108 ml). Note that diary gives the extra details that she leaks with urge, laughing, and running water. Note the caffeine intake.

The ideal duration of the FVC is controversial. The seven-day diary is the most sensitive and accurate, but patients dislike this burden, so compliance is poor. Because the first three days and the last four days of a seven-day test correlate well ($r = 0.9$), most clinicians use a three-day FVC, at least at the first visit. The ICI Committee for Research Methodology found that in most cases, a single 24-hour diary is sufficient. In our Unit, we use a three-day FVC for the first visit, and a 24-hour Urinary Diary for followup visits (see discussion of bladder training in Chapter 7).

THE PAD TEST

The One-Hour Pad Test

This was initially the "industry standard" after its introduction in 1983 and ICS recommendation in 1988. This test involves:

- Patients attend with a comfortably full bladder.
- Are given a pre-weighed continence pad.
- Then drink 500 ml of water over 15 minutes.
- Then perform a standard series of activities to provoke leakage.
- The voided volume is then measured and the wet pad is re-weighed.

Unfortunately, the one-hour pad test fails to correlate with other measures of severity (poor criterion validity) and has poor sensitivity (up to 40% false negative rate). For many years, the one-hour pad test was the only objective method that could be used to define mild (1–10 g leakage per 1 hour), moderate (11–50 g/hr), and severe (>50 g/hr) incontinence; thus it is used in many publications quoted in this text.

The 24-Hour Pad Test

Because of the problems with the 1-hour test, the 24-hour home pad test was developed in the late 1980s. This test involves the following.

- Women are given a set of pre-weighed pads in sealed bags. The pads are worn at home for 24 hours. Ordinary provocative activities are carried out.
- They return pads in a sealed plastic bag, personally or by post, to be re-weighed.

There is no loss of accuracy by evaporation from the sealed plastic bag for durations of 72 hours to two weeks. Thus wet pads can be returned via post. The 24-hour pad test is more sensitive than the 1-hour test (10% false negative rate).

Normal ranges for the 24-hour pad test have been controversial. Studies from 1989–1996 in small samples of women ($n = 23$–78), using simple kitchen scales, gave normal values of 3–8 grams. This seems a lot of fluid on the underwear to be tolerated by an asymptomatic woman. However this definition of "continent" (up to 8 grams) is used throughout most studies in this book.

Recently[6] the normal values were redefined ($n = 120$) using scales accurate to 0.1 g. A median value of 0.3 g (95th centile 1.3 g) was obtained.

The definition of mild, moderate, and severe is important. Because conservative therapy is more likely to cure patients with mild incontinence, and surgery is often offered to patients with severe leakage, a pad test should be able to define severity. Recently mild, moderate, and severe were characterized as 1.3–20 g, 21–74 g, and >75 g on the 24 hour test.[9]

Tests That Measure Anatomical and Functional Observations by Doctors

- The Oxford score for measuring pelvic floor muscle strength and the POPQ scoring system for measuring prolapse were shown in Chapter 2.
- The standard urodynamic test measurements were shown in Chapter 4.

QUALITY OF LIFE

A large array of Quality of Life (QOL) tests have been used in urogynecology.

- Generic tests, that just measure overall QOL, are often used to provide a comparison with other medical therapies (eg cardiac surgery). The SF36 is the most common.
- For incontinence, the two most common are the Urogenital Distress Inventory (UDI) and the Incontinence Impact Questionnaire (IIQ), from the United States. Both come in a short form and have been fully validated. The Kings Health Questionnaire is also often used (from the United Kingdom, available in many languages). For full review see Abrams.[1,2,3]
- In order to perform a health economic analysis, a QOL test that scales from 1–100 needs to be used, such as the York Questionnaire or the AQOL (for review see Hu et al, 2005).

SOCIOECONOMIC EVALUATION

■ A standard test for measuring the personal and treatment costs of incontinence is the Dowell Bryant Incontinence Cost Index (DBICI), which is validated.[4]

■ Another common test is the Willingness to Pay questionnaire, usually tailormade for the particular condition.

CONCLUSIONS

In later chapters in this text, studies that employ validated outcome measures are emphasized, but in the absence of objective data, some studies presenting mainly subjective data are mentioned.

References

1. Abrams P, Khoury S, Wein A, eds (1998) Incontinence: Report of World Health Organisation, 1998; Health, Plymouth UK.
2. Abrams P, Cardozo L, Koury S, Wein A, eds (2001) Incontinence: Report of World Health Organisation, 2001, Health, Plymouth, UK.
3. Abrams P, Cardozo L, Koury S, Wein A, eds (2005) Incontinence: Report of World Health Organisation, 2005, Health, Plymouth, UK.
4. Dowell CJ, Bryant CM, Moore KH, Simons AM (1999) Calculation of the direct costs of urinary incontinence: The DBICI, a new test instrument. Br J Urol 83:596–606.
5. Hu TW, Wagner TH, Hawthorne G, Moore KH, Subak L (2005) Economics of incontinence. In: Abrams P, Cardozo L, Koury S, Wein A (eds). Report of World Health Organisation.
6. Karantanis E, O'Sullivan R, Moore KH (2003) The 24-hour pad test in continent women and men: Normal values and cyclical alterations. Br J Obstet & Gynaecol 110:567–571.
7. Karantanis E, Fynes M, Moore KH, Stanton SL (2004) Comparison of the ICIQ-SF and 24-hour pad test with other measures for evaluating the severity of urodynamic stress incontinence. Int Urogynecol J 15:111–116.
8. Lose G, Fantl A, Victor A, Walter S, Wells T, Wyman J et al (1998) Outcome measures for research in adult women with symptoms of lower urinary tract dysfunction. Neurourol Urodyn 17:255–262.
9. O'Sullivan R, Karantanis E, Stevermuer TL, Allen W, Moore KH (2004) Definition of mild, moderate and severe incontinence on the 24-hour pad test. Br J Obstet Gynaecol 111:859–862.
10. Vaisey C, Garapeti E, Cahill J, Kamm M (1999) Prospective comparison of faecal incontinence grading systems. Gut 44:77–80.

Chapter 6
Conservative Therapy of Urodynamic Stress Incontinence

MANAGING CHRONIC COUGH AND OBESITY

When starting a patient on a conservative treatment program for stress incontinence, you must check whether there are uncorrected precipitating factors.

It is demoralizing for the patient to work hard on a pelvic floor muscle training program if she has uncorrected chronic cough. We often see patients with chronic sinusitis, nasal polyps, post-nasal drip, or asthma/chronic bronchitis, who have never seen an ENT surgeon, or had optimal asthma therapy, and so on.

Many general practitioners have had no training in managing incontinence during their undergraduate years. They may not realize that in the last ten years, enormous advances have been made in conservative continence therapy, but we cannot achieve cure in the presence of an unrelenting cough. Hence sometimes the urogynecologist needs to refer such patients to the appropriate specialist.

Similarly, marked obesity should be reduced whenever possible. Some patients find that when their bodyweight goes over 15–20% overweight, they note stress incontinence, but when they lose weight down below 10–15% overweight, they become continent again. Several objective studies have shown that weight loss reduces stress incontinence.

By striving for reasonable weight loss, you may convert a patient from someone who needs surgery, with the attendant risks in the obese, into a woman who can achieve cure from a conservative program. In our Unit, we do not routinely offer continence surgery to an obese woman without a serious trial of weight loss, because the weight loss may obviate the need for surgery and anesthesia (not to mention the risks of detrusor overactivity and voiding difficulty that come with surgery; see Chapter 9).

Having said this, some obese women are trapped in a vicious circle. They need to exercise in order to lose weight, but whenever they exercise, they leak much more urine than in daily life. In this scenario, we usually strike a deal with the patient. If they can start the process, and lose even 5%, then we will offer surgery if supervised pelvic floor training does not achieve major benefit.

TREATMENT OF CONSTIPATION

Uncorrected constipation (with chronic straining to defecate) is an acknowledged risk factor for stress incontinence. Patients need to learn how to manage this problem before they can expect a conservative program to work.

Further information is provided in Chapter 8 on obstructed defecation, but in essence management is as follows.

- Colorectal surgeons recommend the use of bulking agents such as Metamucil, or psyllium husks (from which Metamucil is manufactured).
- A dessert spoon of psyllium husks should be dissolved in 5–600 ml of water in order to achieve a moist stool that is easily passed.
- A lubricating substance, such as Agarol, can also be introduced, to lubricate the bolus of stool as it moves down the gut.
- In cases where the call to stool is felt, but the bolus of feces cannot be evacuated, then rectal glycerine suppositories are inserted to encourage defecation in this circumstance.
- Regular use of Senekot is now considered unwise, although intermittent doses are helpful if all else fails. Studies by colorectal surgeons indicate that this agent stimulates the nerves of the gut to increase peristalsis and may induce a state of dependence. Eventually the colonic nerves may become refractory.

TREATMENT OF POST-MENOPAUSAL UROGENITAL ATROPHY

We all know that incontinence is more common as age advances, with a peak at the menopause. Because estrogen receptors are known to occur in the urethra, estrogen therapy should give benefit, by thickening the urethral epithelium, improving mucosal coaptation, and enhancing vascular tone in the periurethral vessels.

The Cochrane meta-analysis on use of estrogens for incontinence was last updated in November 2002, and performed an analysis of both systemic and topical estrogen data. They concluded that estrogen has about a 50% benefit for incontinence compared to a 25% benefit for patients on placebo.[19]

Systemic estrogen therapy (HRT) is no longer recommended, as two large trials have recently shown that stress incontinence was worsened in those on HRT compared with those on HRT.[10,14]

The objective benefit of topical vaginal estrogen cream in stress incontinence has received little study. In four small open (nonrandomized, noncontrolled) studies, three showed significant increase in urethral function tests and one showed subjective benefit for continence (20% dry, 55% major benefit). A fifth study showed cure or major benefit on pad testing in 12% of patients versus 0% of controls (for review see Moore[20]).

Practical Advice for Patients

Many elderly women dislike the vaginal applicator that accompanies Oestriol cream (Ovestin). It is cumbersome for those with arthritis, and many do not like inserting the applicator all the way into their vagina and then having to wash it. Some patients stop using it for these reasons (and the first two complaints apply to Vagifem tablets). We encourage patients to put a small amount on their finger and apply it around and just inside the vagina, last thing at night before sleep. Most women find this much more acceptable than using a messy applicator.

STARTING A HOME-BASED PELVIC FLOOR MUSCLE TRAINING PROGRAM

The first step in starting a pelvic floor muscle (PFM) training program should be done during the physical examination (see Figure 6.1). That is, palpate the PFM digitally; make sure the patient can contract the correct muscle.

Discourage her from:

- Contracting the gluteal muscles (lifting buttocks off the bed)
- Contracting the adductor muscles (tightening thighs together)
- Contracting the abdominal muscles (bearing down on the pelvic floor)

Contracting these muscles will not help, and may make leakage worse.

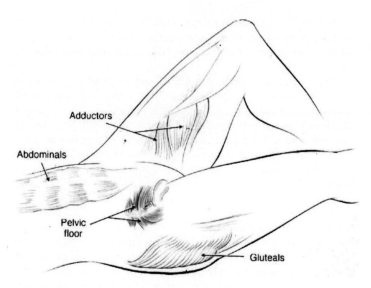

FIGURE 6.1. Assessing the pelvic floor muscles.

Once the patient can contract the PFM correctly, ask her to squeeze as hard as she can, then count up to a maximum of ten seconds. Observe when the muscle starts to fatigue, and stop the count there, for example six seconds.

After the patient has gotten dressed, explain to her that the PFM is a muscle running from the pubic bone to the tail bone, with three openings in it (urethra, vagina, anus). We find it helpful to show a diagram such as that shown in Figure 6.2, inasmuch as many patients don't understand this basic anatomy. Explain that the PFM is a postural muscle, like the erector spinae of the back. Think of the weight lifter who goes to the gymnasium. He usually has a very erect posture because of the strong resting tone of his large back muscles, but he can also lift heavy weights. The woman needs to train her PFM gradually, over 12 to 24 weeks, to increase the resting tone of the muscle, and it will also hypertrophy. Then the patient can train to squeeze the muscle against the "load" of coughing or sneezing.

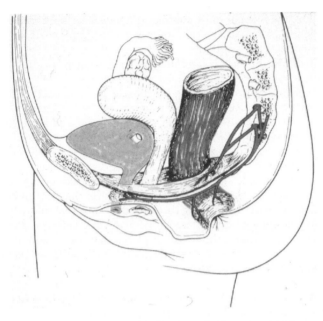

FIGURE 6.2. Diagram of the pelvic floor muscle. (Reprinted with permission from Swash M (1990) The neurogenic hypothesis of stress incontinence. In: Neurobiology of incontinence, No. 151 CIBA Foundation Symposium. John Wiley and Sons, New York, p 160. Copyright 1990, John Wiley & Sons Limited.)

THE ROLE OF THE NURSE CONTINENCE ADVISOR

The assessment and basic explanation of the PFM (as above) is a task that any registrar or clinician should be able to carry out, as it only takes one minute during the physical exam and three or four minutes of explanation time.

The following description of how to start a PFM training program may be too time-consuming within the confines of a busy outpatient clinic. In this case, the patient should be referred to a Nurse Continence Advisor (NCA) for the detailed training given below.

A physiotherapist (physical therapist) will also carry out this type of training program, but in some countries, the NCA is more readily available within a public hospital, with no cost to the patient. Referral to a physiotherapist can therefore be reserved for patients that need electrical stimulation therapy, described later, especially if this incurs a cost.

■ First, the woman must contract the muscle as hard as possible for as long as she can, up to her maximum when fatigue is noted (eg 6 seconds).

■ Then rest the muscle for 5 seconds to let oxygen back into the muscle.

■ Explain that just squeezing the muscle over and over without this oxygen break will cause it to tire out, not strengthen.

■ To make it easy to remember, we usually set a program that builds up numerically from her 6 second maximum, for example 6 second squeeze, 7 squeezes per "set" or group, 8 sets per day.

■ In this example she would perform 56 contractions per day.

■ The 8 sets per day should be spread out over the day, not done all at once in the morning (because this causes fatigue also).

■ To help remember this, we would give 8 red adhesive dots to be placed around the house in places that are visited at different times of the day (near the toothbrush, kettle, telephone, television remote control, etc). See Figure 6.3.

After the patient has strengthened her PFM for three to four weeks, she should then learn how to contract the muscle just before a cough or sneeze. This technique, called "the knack", has been shown on pad testing to reduce leakage by up to 60%/day.[17]

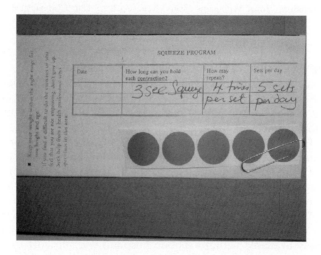

FIGURE 6.3. Written PFM training program for a patient with an initial pelvic floor contraction of only three seconds duration, who is to do four contractions per set, and five sets per day (five red dots given).

In subsequent visits, the nurse continence advisor reiterates the initial explanation and upgrades the program (makes it harder). If a patient is sent to physiotherapy, the first visit always includes this type of explanation, with upgrading at followup. Even if the main complaint is urge incontinence, the PFM is used to defer micturition, so patients need to know how to contract it.

WHO SHOULD BE REFERRED FOR PHYSIOTHERAPY?

If a woman cannot contract her PFM at the initial examination (or can only manage a weak flicker) despite your best efforts to help her locate the muscle, then she definitely needs referral to a pelvic floor physiotherapist (a physiotherapist who has undergone subspecialty training). She will assess the patient vaginally, use additional methods to help her identify the muscle, then move on to biofeedback or electrostimulation or both (see below for details).

The question then becomes, do women who can contract their muscles need a supervised training program, or can they practice at home with equally good results? This leads into the question: What form of PFM training is most effective?

In the last 25 years, many publications have considered this question. One problem is that the outcome measures used by the different authors varied greatly. Table 6.1 summarizes the results. The term "hospital PFMT" indicates that patients attended a pelvic floor physiotherapist or nurse continence advisor weekly or monthly and had regular supervision of their training program.

The duration of followup in these various trials also varied a great deal. Nevertheless it can be seen that supervised PFM training yields generally higher success rates (average about 50% cure, range 25–75%), compared to a home-based program (29% cure).

Another problem with this table of results is that the severity of leakage at baseline was seldom taken into account. Stratified randomization was rare (so that mild and severe patients could be distributed equally into both treatment arms). A study in which only patients with mild to moderate incontinence (on one-hour pad test) were recruited (with stratified randomization) showed that 65% of those with mild incontinence were cured, compared to a 35% cure rate for moderate incontinence.[20] In this pragmatic trial, only patients with a weak pelvic floor were referred for electrostimulation: the cost was not

TABLE 6.1. Objective Results After Pelvic Floor Muscle Training for Stress Incontinence

Authors	N	Treatment	Results
Wilson et al (1987)	15	Home PFME	Pads/24 hours 11% benefit
	45	Hospital PFME	Pads/24 hours 54% benefit
Jolleys (1989)	65	Home PFME	48% subjectively dry
	56	Control	0% subjectively dry
Henalla et al (1989)	25	Hospital PFME	65% cure/ marked benefit pad test
	24	Control	0% cure/marked benefit pad test
Burns et al (1990)	38	Hospital PFME	54% reduction leaks/wk FVC
	40	Control	9% worse leaks/wk FVC
Ramsay and Thou (1990)	22	Home PFME	1.5 g worse on 1 hr pad test
	22	Control-contract thighs	2.1 g better on 1 hr pad test
Bo et al (1990)	26	Home PFME	Pad test change NS
	26	Hospital PFME	Pad test 27 g fell to 7.1 g/hr
Bo et al (1995)	23	Hospital PFME	75% dry on urodynamic cough test at 5 yrs
Wells et al (1991)	82	Hospital PFME	27% dry on wetting diary
	75	Phenylpropanolamine	14% dry on wetting diary
Mouritsen et al (1991)	100	Hospital PFME	47% dry pad test at 12 months
Cammu et al (1991)	52	Hospital PFME	25% dry on FVC
O'Brien et al (1991)	292	Home PFME	29% no longer using pads
	132	Control	No benefit
Lagro-Janssen et al (1992)	53	Home PFME	Leaks/wk 19.6, fell to 7.2/wk
	57	Control	Leaks/wk 21, worse, to 23/wk
Hahn et al (1993)	170	Hospital PFME	35% dry on stress test
	30	Control	0% change in controls
Seim et al (1996)	96	Hospital PFME	48-hour pad test 28 g fell to 10 g
Bo et al (1999)	25	Hospital PFME	44% dry, pad test at 6 mos
	30	Control	6% dry, pad test at 6 mos

felt to be warranted in those with a good contraction strength at baseline.

A meta-analysis[1] and a recent Cochrane Collaboration meta-analysis[12] both emphasized poor standardization of outcome measures and followup duration, but concluded that PFM training is clearly superior to no treatment, and a supervised program gives better results than a home-based program.

WHAT DOES THE PHYSIOTHERAPIST DO THAT INCREASES EFFICACY?

Basically the pelvic floor physiotherapist has three techniques:

- To act as a personal trainer, just as for an athlete
  —To re-examine the PFM at regular intervals to check strength and increase the difficulty of the training program
  —To evaluate the frequency volume chart with the patient regularly; see whether leakage is really declining
  —To remind the patient to perform "the knack" as they often forget
  —To increase motivation by positive verbal feedback (as results improve)
- To use some form of "biofeedback" technique such as
  —A graduated perineometer, to show contraction strength (Figure 6.4)
  —Verbal biofeedback during digital examination, asking the patient to contract harder or for a longer duration
  —Vaginal weighted cones, that the patient wears in the vagina for 20 minutes twice daily, with steady increase in the cone weights (Figure 6.5)
  —Mechanical or auditory biofeedback, such as a vaginal pressure transducer that conveys increased pressure by an increased auditory or visual signal
- To employ electrostimulation therapy when the patient has a weak or absent PFM contraction, which may comprise
  —Trans-vaginal electrostimulation, also called faradism (Figure 6.6)
  —Trans-suprapubic electrostimulation, or interferential therapy

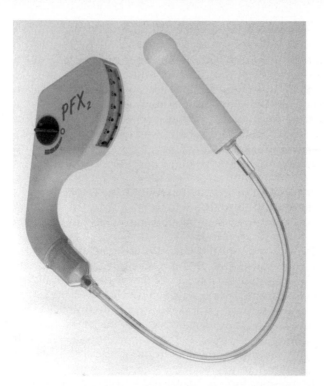

FIGURE 6.4. Perineometer. Used to measure strength of the PFM contraction. (Reprinted with permission from Moore KH (2000) Conservative therapy for incontinence. In: Balliere's Clinical Obstetrics and Gynaecology, ed. Cardozo L. 14:251–289; Copyright 2000, Elsevier.)

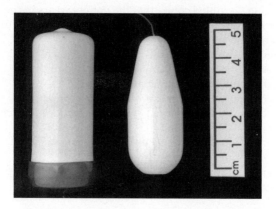

FIGURE 6.5. Vaginal cones. Used to teach patients how to contract the PFM. (Reprinted with permission from Moore KH (2000) Conservative therapy for incontinence. In: Balliere's Clinical Obstetrics and Gynaecology, ed. Cardozo L. 14:251–289; Copyright 2000, Elsevier.)

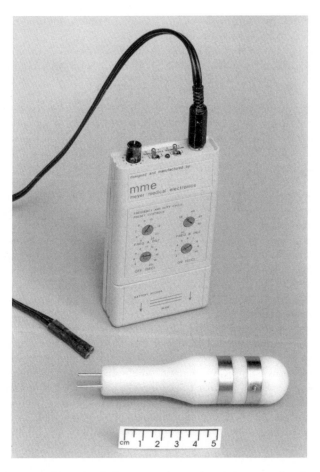

FIGURE 6.6. Intravaginal electrostimulation device. (Reprinted with permission from Moore KH (2000) Conservative therapy for incontinence. In: Balliere's Clinical Obstetrics and Gynaecology, ed. Cardozo L. 14:268–272; Copyright 2000, Elsevier.)

THE EFFICACY OF PHYSIOTHERAPY TECHNIQUES

For a detailed analysis of this issue, the reader should consult a dedicated text, such as *Pelvic Floor Re-education*.[24] Nevertheless, some conclusions can be made. The first item of physiotherapy training above (acting as a personal trainer to enhance performance and gradually increase the difficulty of the training) is clearly efficacious, as shown in Table 6.1 regarding home training versus supervised training.

Biofeedback is quite controversial. The following statements are evidence-based. In a compact book such as this, it is not practical to cite all evidence.

Use of the *perineometer* aids the patient by measuring the degree of improvement in pelvic floor muscle strength. This does not always translate into improved continence, unless the patient uses her PFM during cough or other episodes of raised intra-abdominal pressure (the knack).

Use of *vaginal weighted cones* provides a variable degree of enhanced efficacy. In some studies they give major benefit; in other studies the benefit over PFM training is not statistically significant. The Cochrane meta-analysis found no clearly significant overall benefit from their use. We find that a patient's attitude towards a self-inserted vaginal device is very important. Some women find them a useful aid; others cannot accept the idea of inserting a cone into their vagina. They are "another option" for women having difficulty with simple PFM training who do not want surgery.

Use of *auditory or visual biofeedback* techniques to enhance the woman's appreciation of her PFM strength is controversial. Most studies do not contain adequate numbers to show significant benefit. Such devices are often quite expensive, so that for the ordinary clinician, a major benefit needs to be shown before the cost outlay is worthwhile. Some physiotherapists use biofeedback at the first visit to help women identify their PFM, but don't always use it at followup visits.[9]

Use of electrostimulation is physiologically attractive. The skeletal muscle of the PFM is given a regular electrical stimulus, which causes a tetanic (maximal strength) contraction. In our experience, electrostimulation is very useful for the woman who simply cannot contract her PFM at the first visit. Once she can feel it contracting, she should be given a detailed PFM training program to use between the electrostimulation visits. Unfortunately, most studies of this technique do not specifically select women who are unable to contract the PFM, and do not give a PFM training program for use between electrostimulation visits. Most of the studies are very small ($n = 20–30$ in either arm), so that they are "underpowered" to achieve a significant result. Partly this is because the studies are "purist"; ie they do not allow a PFM program to be utilized. Therefore it is difficult to recruit patients into these studies.

The World Health Organization concluded that "There is insufficient evidence to judge whether electrical stimulation is better than no treatment for women with urodynamic stress incontinence."[28]

Extra-Corporeal Electromagnetic Stimulation Therapy
This is an alternative form of electrostimulation therapy that avoids the need for a vaginal probe. Patients sit fully clothed on a chair that contains a magnetic coil under the seat. Preliminary studies show promising results.[8]

WHAT TO DO IF CONSERVATIVE THERAPY FAILS BUT PATIENT DOES NOT WANT SURGERY
Prior to the 1990s such patients were left with the main option of using continence pads. In the last decade, several bioengineering companies have taken up the challenge to develop mechanical devices that can correct incontinence.

The first of these was the bladder neck support prosthesis (Introl, Figure 6.7), which is shaped like a prolapse ring pessary but has two prongs that sit in the retropubic space and cradle the urethra. Clinical trials indicate that 62% of those who can be fitted become continent (see Moore[19]). The device is difficult to

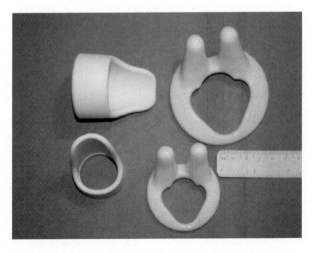

FIGURE 6.7. Contiform (left side) and Introl (right side) devices.

fit in those with multiple previous failed continence surgery, but is well suited to those without previous surgery who mainly leak during sporting activities. It is also useful for patients with co-existent prolapse. At present it is available in Japan and Australia.

The same inventor went on to develop a simpler device, Contiform, that is shaped like a hollow tampon (Figure 6.7). Initially this device was only available in three sizes, and gave a highly significant reduction in incontinence, but the "cure" rate on pad testing was only 22% (Morris et al[21]). Subsequently a fourth size has been manufactured; clinical trials are ongoing. This device does not treat prolapse, but is useful in patients who mainly leak with sporting activities and do not want surgery.

CONCLUSIONS
PFM training needs to be tailored to the individual woman. Stress incontinence is not life threatening, and patients know this. Do not recommend a therapy that the patient feels uncomfortable with, as her compliance will be poor. In order to provide the best results, discuss the options with the patient, and let her select that with which she thinks she can comply.

The caveat to this advice is that patients should also understand the risks of surgery, should they not respond to conservative therapy. If a woman understands that current continence surgery has a 5–6% risk of developing overactive bladder, and a 1–2% risk of voiding difficulty, then their interest in and compliance with conservative therapy may be enhanced. Urogynecologists must always remember that our first duty is "to do no harm," and PFM training has no complications.

References
1. Berghmans LC, Hendriks HJ, Bo K et al (1998) Conservative treatment of genuine stress incontinence in women: A systematic review of randomized clinical trials Brit J Urol 82:181–191.
2. Bo K, Hagen RH, Kvarstein B, Jorgensen J, Larson S (1990) Pelvic floor muscle exercise for treatment of female stress urinary incontinence. III: Effects of two different degrees of pelvic floor muscle exercises. Neurourol Urodyn 9:489–502.
3. Bo K, Talseth T (1995) Five year follow up of pelvic floor muscle exercise for treatment of stress urinary incontinence, Clinical and urodynamic assessment. Neurourol Urodyn 14:374–376.
4. Bo K, Talseth T, Holme I (1999) Single blind randomized controlled trial of pelvic floor exercises, electrical stimulation, vaginal cones, and no treatment in management of genuine stress incontinence in women. BMJ 318:487–493.

5. Burns P, Pranikoff K, Nochajski M, Desotelle P, Harwood M (1990) Treatment of stress incontinence with pelvic floor exercises and biofeedback. J Am Geriatr Soc 38:341–344.

6. Cammu H, Van Hylen M, Derde MP, Debruyne R, Amy JJ (1991) Pelvic physiotherapy in genuine stress incontinence. Urology 38:332–337.

7. Fantl JA, Cardozo L, McClish DK, and the Hormones and Urogenital Therapy Committee (1994) Estrogen therapy in the management of urinary incontinence in postmenopausal women: A meta-analysis. Obstet Gynecol 83:12–18.

8. Goldberg RP, Galloway NT, Sand PK (2004) Extracorporeal electromagnetic stimulation therapy, In: Bourcier AP, McGuire EJ, Abrams P (eds) Pelvic floor disorders, Elsevier Saunders, Philadelphia, Chapter 30, pp 291–296.

9. Goode PS, Burgio KL, Locher JL et al (2003) Effect of behavioural training with or without pelvic floor electrical stimulation on stress in continence in women. A randomixed controlled trial. JAMA 290:345–352.

10. Grady D, Brown JS, Vittinghoff E (2001) HERS Research Group. Postmenopausal hormones and incontinence; the Heart and Estrogen/Progestin Replacement Study. Obstet Gynecol 97:116–120.

11. Hahn I, Milson J, Fall M, Eklund P (1993) Long term results of pelvic floor training in female stress urinary incontinence. Br J Urol 72:421–427.

12. Hay-Smith EJ, Bo Berghmns LC, Hendriks HJ, de Bie RA, van Waalwijk van Doorn ES (2001) Pelvic floor muscle training for urinary incontinence in women. Cochrane Database Systematic Review 1:DC001407.

13. Henalla SM, Hutchins CJ, Robinson P, MacVicar J (1989) Nonoperative methods in the treatment of female genuine stress incontinence of urine. J Obstet Gynecol 9:222–225.

14. Jackson RA, Vittinghof E, Kanaya AM et al (2004) Urinary incontinence in elderly women: Findings from the Health Aging and Body Composition Study. Obstet Gynecol 104:301–307.

15. Jolleys J (1989) Diagnosis and management of female urinary incontinence in general practice. J Roy Coll Gen Pract 39:277–279.

16. Lagro Janssen ALM, Debruyne FMJ, Smits AJA, Van Weel C (1992) The effects of treatment of urinary incontinence in general practice. Fam Pract 9:284–289.

17. Miller J, Aston-Miller JA, DeLancey JOL (1996) The knack: Use of precisely timed pelvic muscle contraction can reduce leakage in SUI. Neurourol Urodyn 15:392–393.

18. Moehrer B et al (2003) Oestrogens for urinary incontinence (Review) Cochrane database. CD001405.DOI: 10.1002/14651858.CD.

19. Moore KH (2000) Conservative therapy for incontinence. In: Balliere's Clinical Obstetrics and Gynaecology, ed. Cardozo, L. 14:251–289.

20. Moore KH, O'Sullivan RJ, Simons A, Prashar S, Anderson P, Louey M (2003) Randomized controlled trial of nurse continence advisor

therapy versus standard urogynaecology regime for conservative incontinence treatment: Efficacy, costs and two year follow up. Brit J Obstet Gynaecol 110:649–657.

21. Morris A, Moore KH (2003) The contiform incontinence device— efficacy and patient acceptibility. Int J Urogynaecology 14:412–417.

22. O'Brien J, Austin M, Sethi P, O'Boyle P (1991) Urinary incontinence: Prevalence, need for treatment, and effectiveness of intervention by nurse. Br Med J 303:1308–1312.

23. Ramsay IN, Thou M (1990) A randomised double blind placebo controlled trial of pelvic floor exercises in the treatment of genuine stress incontinence. Neurourol Urodyn 9:398–399.

24. Schuessler B, Norton PA, Stanton SL, et al. Pelvic Floor Reeducation: Principles and Practice, second edition. Springer Verlag London Ltd, 2006 (in press).

25. Seim A, Siversen B, Eriksen BC, Hunskar S (1996) Treatment of urinary incontinence in women in general practice: An observational study. Br Med J 312:1459–1462.

26. Wells TJ, Brink MPH, Diokno AC, Wolfe R, Gillis GL (1991) Pelvic muscle exercise for stress urinary incontinence in elderly women. J Am Geriatr Soc 39:785–791.

27. Wilson PD, Al Samarrai T, Deakein M, Kolbe E, Brown ADG (1987) An objective assessment of physiotherapy for female genuine stress incontinence. Br Obstet and Gynaecol 94:575–582.

28. Wilson PD, Hay Smith J, Nygaard J et al (2005) Adult conservative management. In: Abrams P, Cardoza L, Khoury S, Wein A (eds) Incontinence, Report of 3rd International Consultation on Incontinence. Health Publications Ltd, Plymouth, pp 855–964.

Chapter 7

Step-by-Step Guide to Treatment of Overactive Bladder (OAB)/ Detrusor Overactivity

If a patient has pure frequency/urgency/nocturia/urge incontinence symptoms on history, or if urodynamic testing has revealed detrusor overactivity, then bladder training is an essential part of treatment.

EXPLAIN THE CONDITION

This is the first step. Many patients with this problem think that they are "neurotic"; often they are an embarrassment to their families as they frequently need to rush to the toilet at social occasions. In fact, during the 1970s and 1980s, several studies were undertaken to support the theory that this condition was largely psychosomatic, but conclusive evidence of this was not found.

Since the introduction of quality of life testing in the 1990s, we have learned that patients with detrusor overactivity have a much poorer quality of life than those with stress incontinence, and are more anxious and depressed because of the unpredictable nature of their condition.

Recent studies have indicated that

- The subepithelial nerves are overabundant in this condition (increased by about 35%;[19] see Figure 7.1), and neuropeptides involved in conveying "nociceptive" or painful symptoms are increased by 80–90%.[27]
- The ability of the cerebral cortex to inhibit the desire to void is reduced in this condition, but can be strengthened by training.
- The detrusor muscle is overly contractile, giving rise to "muscle cramps" in the bladder. Pharmacological studies

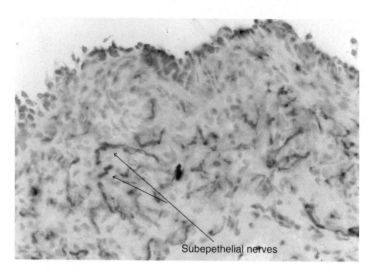

Subepethelial nerves

FIGURE 7.1. Increased subepithelial nerves in detrusor overactivity patient.

show that, in the organ bath, the muscle strips from these patients do not relax entirely when atropine is administered (whereas detrusor strips from control patients do relax after atropine is applied). (For review see Kumar.[17])

Therefore the patient must understand that she is not neurotic, but has an abnormality of the afferent (subepithelial nerves) and efferent (detrusor contractility) limbs of the micturition reflex.

The next step in bladder training is to look at the Frequency Volume Chart with the patient. Because severity of frequency varies in this condition, the therapist needs to find a realistic target "voiding interval" towards which the patient can aim. For example if the chart shows that the patient usually toilets every hour, but sometimes can hold for two hours, then the target voiding interval should be two hours (Figure 7.2).

Once the target (eg two hours) is chosen, the instructions to the patient are as follows.

STEP-BY-STEP GUIDE TO BLADDER TRAINING

When you get a desire to go to the toilet, look at your
watch.

If it is more than two hours since you last went to the toilet,
just go ahead and pass urine.

If it is less than two hours since you last went, then you
need to do three things:

    A. Sit down.

        The reason for this is that the bladder has gravity
nerves inside the wall, that give you a stronger
desire to toilet when you are standing than when
you are sitting.

    B. Contract your pelvic floor muscle (PFM).

        The reason is that you must stop any drops of urine
escaping from your bladder into your urethra.
Once the fluid gets into your urethra, there is an
automatic reflex that will make you start passing
urine onto your pad, so you need to "nip this in
the bud."

    C. Send a strong message from your brain, down your
spinal cord to the level of the tailbone, then out to
your bladder, saying, "*No*, I am *not* going to the
toilet for 2 minutes."

        There is a direct pathway from the front of your brain,
down the spine, to the bladder, but in your condition the message signals on this pathway seem to
have become "rusty" or weak. These messages can
be strengthened by focused concentration.

Sit quietly for two minutes, contracting your PFM. At the
end of two minutes,

Stand up (contracting your PFM as you stand) and walk
slowly to the toilet (do not run or you are more likely
to leak).

However, if you have waited two minutes,

It is likely that YOU WILL NO LONGER WANT TO GO.

This is because the bladder spasms that cause your leakage
are like a muscle cramp; they normally only last 1–2
minutes and then the muscle can't hold the spasm any
more; it relaxes.

Therefore you may be able to hold on for another half an hour
or so, until another spasm occurs. If this happens after
you have successfully stopped the previous spasm, then
you should go ahead and walk to the toilet for this one.

	TIME AND VOLUME RECORD Please fill in the chart for the number of days specified by the Continence Advisor, noting carefully the required information.				MRN SURNAME OTHER NAMES DOB 15·9·36 SEX F AMO	
					Affix Addressograph Label here	
DATE	TIME	INTERVAL	VOLUME	LEAKAGE	BOWELS OPENED	FLUID INTAKE
Example 27.4.99	9 am		200 ml	SMALL YES	YES	1 CUP TEA
	11 am	2 Hrs	150 ml	NO	NO	1 GLASS H2O, 1 CUP TEA
23·9·01	5·30 am	7½ HRS	500 ml	NO	NO	1 GLASS H2O
	7·30 am	2 HR	200 ml	YES	NO	Good! ✱
	8·00 am	½ HR	100 ml	NO	YES	No!
	9·15 am	1½ HRS	300 ml	A LOT FRONT DOOR	NO	2 GLASS H2O
	10·45 am	1½ HRS	250 ml	NO	NO	1 " "
	11·50 am	1 HR 5 MIN	230 ml	NO	NO	1 " " No!
	1·10 pm	1 HR 20 MIN	250 ml	NO	YES	
	2·55 pm	1 HR 45 MIN	200 ml	YES	NO	2 " "
	4·45 pm	1 HR 50 MIN	280 ml	NO	NO	Good! ✱
	5·55 pm	1 HR 10 MIN	300 ml	NO	NO	1 " "
	10·25 pm	5 HRS 30 MIN	270 ml	NO	NO	Great !!

FIGURE 7.2. A typical example of a patient with OAB, with the usual voiding frequency circled, and the "target" voiding interval underlined.

Before the patient can successfully undertake Step B, she must be examined to make sure that she can contract her PFM, and if not, undergo a program of pelvic floor muscle training, as described in Chapter 6. Do not disappoint the patient by expecting her to succeed with bladder training until she has learned how to contract the pelvic floor muscle.

The patient needs to understand that bladder training is an essential part of treating the overactive bladder. If drugs are prescribed for this condition, they will help to relax the bladder spasms, but the patient must try to inhibit the premature desire to void. Also, if a patient suffers from nocturia, the bladder training works to increase her bladder capacity during the day. Gradually, her bladder capacity will also increase at night. She must attempt to inhibit the desire to void at night if she is awakened by a snoring husband or a dog that is barking. She must avoid nocturnal trips to the toilet out of habit.

HOW DO ANTICHOLINERGIC DRUGS WORK AND HOW DO WE USE THEM?

Anticholinergic drugs work through the parasympathetic nervous system; they are antagonists that work at the muscarinic receptor to inhibit (and in some cases abolish) detrusor muscle contractions. For the patient, this can be likened to a muscle relaxant acting on the bladder. There are several types of anticholinergic drugs, some of which have additional pharmacological properties.

Propantheline (Probanthine): 15 mg TDS is a very old antimuscarinic drug that was initially used for gastric ulcers. Its structure (quaternary amine) means that it is poorly absorbed from the gut. Side effects of dry mouth and constipation are almost always experienced, but the drug is cheap.

Oxybutynin (Ditropan): Maximum 5 mg TDS has been used since the 1970s. It acts as an antimuscarinic drug, but also has local anesthetic properties (thus it can be given intra-vesically), and also a smooth muscle relaxation effect. It is very effective in reducing detrusor contractions, but about 60% of patients will get annoying dry mouth/dryness of the esophagus/difficulty swallowing and stop taking it. It is also very cheap. When giving oxybutynin, titrate the dose against the symptoms. For severe nocturia but less daytime leak, give 2.5 mg mane and 5 mg nocte. Some patients are worse in the morning but have no nocturia; give 5 mg mane and 2.5 mg after lunch. The drug works within one hour and lasts six to eight hours. A long-acting "slow release" form of oxybutynin has been developed but is not marketed in some countries; this gives less dry mouth (about 25%). A trans-dermal patch is also made, but gives pruritis at the patch site in about 7% of patients and is not yet widely available.

Imipramine (Tofranil): 10 mg mane, 20 mg nocte is also a very old drug. In much larger doses (75–100 mg daily) it is an antidepressant. It has a Beta-mimetic action to relax the dome of the bladder, but also has anticholinergic effects. Because a common side effect is drowsiness, it is very useful for nocturia. It also lowers the pain threshold by an uncertain mechanism, and can be used when the bladder spasms are appreciated as painful (or in painful bladder syndrome; see Chapter 12).

Tolteridine (Detrusitol): 2 mg BD was developed in the 1990s. It attaches to the bladder muscarinic receptors to a much greater extent than to such receptors in the salivary glands, so it gives less dry mouth than oxybutynin but is just as effective. It also has a slightly longer duration of effect; hence the BD dosage. In some patients, 4 mg BD can be given without dry mouth. It is available in most countries now (although only as a "private" prescription in Australia; thus it is expensive, AU\$ 55–80 per month). A slow release form has been made which is somewhat more effective with even less dry mouth, but is not available in all countries.

Propiverine (Detrunorm): 15 mg TDS is an antimuscarinic agent that is also a calcium channel blocker. Some women who do not respond to any of the above drugs will respond to this agent, as if there is an individual response. Dry mouth occurs in about 20% of patients but is not usually distressing. It is not available in many countries.

Trospium: 20 mg BD is a nonselective quaternary amine, but does not give as much dry mouth (4%). Its structure also limits blood–brain barrier penetration, thus reducing CNS effects in the elderly (confusion). It is widely used in the United Kingdom.

Darifenacin: Selectively acts at the M3 receptor, which is thought to be most functionally important for mediating detrusor contractions. Unfortunately it was developed in the late 1990s but not marketed for commercial reasons.

Solifenacin: 5–10 mg daily is also selective for the M3 receptor and also does not attach well to the salivary gland receptors. It was developed in early 2000s and achieved continence in 51% of one trial, with 11% suffering from dry mouth. At present it is only available in a few countries.

Duloxetine: An additional new agent, this is a serotonin re-uptake inhibitor that also affects Oluf's nucleus in the pelvic nerve plexus. It was designed for the medical treatment of stress incontinence because it enhances the strength of the internal urethral sphincter mechanism. Because it also enhances bladder capacity, it has also been used in overactive bladder. It has obtained European approval and is available in Denmark.

Desmopressin (Minirin): Consider treating with this if nocturia is a major problem. This synthetic vasopressin analogue markedly reduces the production of urine for about six hours. It is given as a one nasal spray to each nostril before bedtime. It is useful for patients with debilitating nocturia who are practicing bladder training during the day but have not yet improved their bladder capacity, so they have not yet seen any reduction in nocturia. It is not a good long-term strategy. Particularly in the elderly, prolonged use is associated with hyponatremia that can be life threatening. Beware the patient with nocturnal polyuria, however (defined as passing more than 30% of total urine output at night). This drug is contraindicated in such patients so a frequency volume chart *must* be completed before starting this drug. In children with bedwetting, long-term usage has been shown to be safe.

ARE ANTICHOLINERGIC DRUGS EFFECTIVE?

This is highly controversial. Most pharmacotherapy trials only consider efficacy at 12 weeks or thereabouts. A recent Cochrane meta-analysis[16] found that, in a review of 6713 patients in 51 studies, the placebo effect was much higher than expected (about 45% with respect to control), but that the drugs gave an additional 15% over placebo. Overall, anticholinergic drugs achieved one less leak per 48 hours and one less void per 48 hours, with respect to placebo. This may seem like a small effect, but most of these trials did not include formal bladder training programs, so they do not reflect ordinary clinical practice.

The natural history of detrusor overactivity has received little attention. Recently a review of 76 patients with proven DO at a median of six years[21] found that symptoms had largely resolved in only about 16%. Symptoms were no different in 59% of patients, and were worse in the remaining 25% (Figure 7.3). Thus

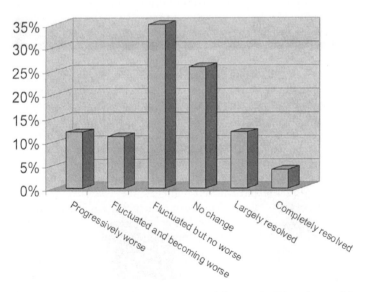

FIGURE 7.3. Histogram showing course of disease in 76 patients with detrusor overactivity at a median followup of six years (data from Morris et al[21]).

some form of long-term anticholinergic therapy may be needed in up to three quarters of patients.

Having said that, patients may not have to take the full dose to achieve good symptom control. Many patients have "good days" and "bad days". In a randomized controlled trial, Burton[7] showed that patients who took tablets only on their "bad days" (the "PRN regime") obtained equally good effect as those who took the daily dose.

ROLE OF TOPICAL ESTROGENS

Theoretically, the effect of vaginal estrogen upon the bladder base/trigone should promote tissue elasticity and enhance bladder capacity. Also the effects of estrogen seen in patients with stress incontinence (thickening the urethral mucosa to prevent leakage of urine) should also help to reduce leakage in women with OAB.

Unfortunately, few studies have investigated this. Small studies from the early 1980s showed significant improvement in urge incontinence symptoms, but no objective outcome parameters were employed. A large RCT of topical estrogen versus placebo showed no significant benefit for urge symptoms, but the dose of estrogen was found to be insufficient when the effect of estrogen upon the cytopathology of urethral epithelial swabs was fully evaluated.[3]

ALTERNATIVE THERAPIES FOR DETRUSOR OVERACTIVITY

TENS (Trans-Cutaneous Electrostimulation Therapy)

This has been used for many years in the labor ward, to inhibit the sensation of pain during uterine contractions. TENS (Figure 7.4) has been applied with some success in patients who feel the urge to void as a painful spasm. It works by modifying sensory input, by interrupting the relay of afferent impulses to the cerebral cortex (called the gateway theory of pain control).

The electrodes are applied over the pubic bone or over the sacrum, and the patient self-regulates the electrical impulses coming from the stimulator (worn attached to her belt) until she feels a strong buzzing or throbbing sensation over the application site. Small clinical trials have shown promising results.[5,14] The device costs about 50 Euros.

Acupuncture

Acupuncture has also been helpful for detrusor overactivity. Initially it was thought to work via the gateway theory of pain con-

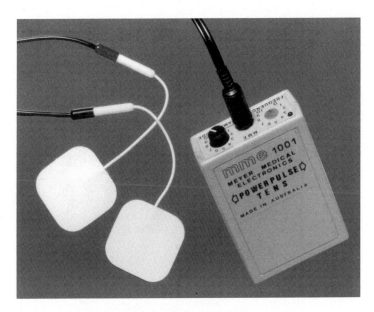

FIGURE 7.4. TENS machine for the treatment of detrusor overactivity. (Reprinted with permission from Moore KH (2000) Conservative therapy for incontinence. In: Arulkumaran S (ed) Clin Obstet Gynaecol 14:279; Copyright, 2000, Elsevier.)

trol, but later it was found that acupuncture increases the levels of endogenous opioids (beta-endorphin and met-enkephalin) in the patient's cerebrospinal fluid. Pharmacological experiments show that enkephalins inhibit detrusor contractions.

The traditional bladder points are documented in the literature; in one small study[22] ($n = 16$), acupuncture abolished detrusor overactivity incontinence in 63%. In a larger study ($n = 26$ patients on active acupuncture, 24 sham therapy), symptom improvement occurred in 85%, with 75% becoming urodynamically stable.[8]

SANS Electro-Acupuncture (Stoller Afferent Nerve Stimulator)

This is a device that mimics acupuncture, but adds an electrical stimulus to the needle that is inserted into a bladder point over the medial malleolus of the ankle (near the posterior tibial nerve). This device can be employed by trained nurse continence advisors, because the relevant bladder point is easily identified from surface anatomy (Figure 7.5) Acute administration of SANS

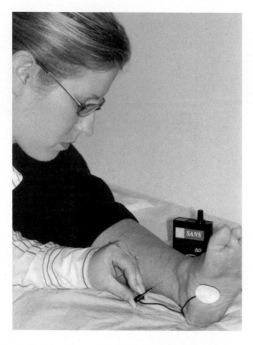

FIGURE 7.5. SANS device, applied to the bladder acupuncture point at the medial malleolus.

during cystometry significantly increased the volume at first detrusor contraction and the maximum cystometric capacity.[1] After 12 weeks of SANS in 53 patients, a 25% reduction in frequency, 21% reduction in nocturia, and a 35% benefit for urge incontinence were noted.[13]

Hypnotherapy

Hypnotherapy has also been helpful.[11] After one month of 12 sessions, 58% of 63 patients became symptom free; 14% were unchanged. Cystometry showed that 50% had become stable, with 36% improved. Of 30 patients reviewed at two years, 33% remained symptom free. The author commented that patients required an audiocassette tape to be used in their own homes at regular intervals in order to maintain symptomatic benefit, so this therapy requires a dedicated user.

Electrostimulation

As discussed in Chapter 6, electrostimulation is a recognized technique for strengthening the pelvic floor muscle, by inducing repetitive tetanic muscle contractions. It can also be used for patients with detrusor overactivity (DO). Electrostimulation of the nerves of the perineum or anus is known to cause reflex inhibition of detrusor contractions. In the 1970s, electrostimulation was usually delivered via an anal electrode, which was not popular among middle-aged women. More recently, Brubaker et al[6] showed that intra-vaginal electrostimulation resulted in a urodynamically stable bladder in 49% of patients with DO (no significant change in the sham group).

Extra-Corporeal Electromagnetic Stimulation Therapy

As mentioned in Chapter 6, this is a form of electrostimulation therapy that avoids the need for a vaginal probe. "On-chair" cystometry studies show that the magnetic coil stimulus abolishes detrusor overactivity in the majority of cases, but results of long-term clinical treatment are awaited. (For review see Goldberg et al[12] and Morris[20]).

Cystodistension

Originally Helmstein's cystodistension was undertaken for five to seven hours (under epidural anesthesia) in order to produce necrosis of superficial bladder tumors. Later studies showed that this degree of distension produced tissue anoxia, which was thought to reduce detrusor contractility. Studies in the 1970s showed subjective response for DO in 70%, with 65–80% of bladders becoming urodynamically stable.[23] Later studies showed symptomatic response in 32%, with a stable bladder in 19%.[10] These days it is difficult to justify epidural anesthesia and day-only admission for such a response rate.

However, in patients over age 50 with refractory detrusor overactivity (defined as failure to respond to two anticholinergic drugs with bladder training for more than 12 months,[19]) it is reasonable to offer cystoscopy to exclude carcinoma in situ (which may cause chronic irritative symptoms eg frequency, urgency, and nocturia) and at the same time perform a simple cystodistension. This involves distending the bladder to capacity under general anesthetic, then allowing the total fluid volume to remain in the bladder for three to five minutes (with the infusion bag at a height of one meter above the bladder). A refill examination can then be performed in patients who also complain of suprapubic pain (see Chapter 12) to exclude interstitial cystitis.

Clam Cystoplasty

This was popular in the 1980s. In patients with completely refractory disease, the bladder was opened transversely (in the manner of opening a clam) and a segment of flattened bowel was inserted into the bladder opening, then the bladder was closed with its interposed bowel segment in continuity. The idea was to increase the bladder capacity, and interpose an autologous tissue that would impair detrusor muscle contractility.

This procedure has a 1% mortality rate, and the initial 90% subjective response was not sustained over time. The bladder becomes stable in about 60% of cases. At a mean followup of six years,[2] 53% of 51 patients were continent but 40% needed to self-catheterize and suffered recurrent UTI. Mucous plugs from the bowel segment caused urinary retention in 20%.

Partial Detrusor Myomectomy

The concerns about risks versus benefits for the clam cystoplasty procedure led to its development.[18,28] It yields better results with less morbidity.

Implantation of S3 Sacral Nerve Root Stimulator

A two-stage procedure that can be effective for refractory DO, it is very expensive and requires careful followup of the patient. The first stage involves Peripheral Nerve Evaluation (PNE). Under local anesthetic, with the patient lying prone, the S3 foramen is located, a spinal needle is used to test that the nerve root has been located by electrical stimulation, and then a temporary stimulation wire is inserted and taped securely. This is attached to a temporary pulse generator device that the patient wears externally. The patient goes home for five to seven days, and records the impact of the S3 stimulation upon their DO symptoms. If the symptomatic benefit after PNE is greater than 50–70%, a permanent electrode is implanted into the S3 foramen and secured by nonabsorbable sutures to the periosteum. The pulse generator is then implanted in a pouch, inside the anterior superior iliac crest. Early results[4] and long-term followup[25,26] indicate that the frequency and severity of urge incontinence episodes is substantially reduced (see Hassouna[15] for review).

Botox Therapy (Botulinim Toxin A Injections)

These injections to the detrusor muscle have recently been used in neuropathic DO, and limited trials have been performed in idiopathic DO. The neurotoxin binds to cholinergic terminals locally to inhibit acetylcholine release, resulting in paralysis at the injected muscle site. It also blocks the release of some afferent neuropeptides involved in transmission of noxious stimuli. About 30 injections are usually given, via cystoscopy. Botox has been widely used in neuropathic DO with objective benefit in urodynamic outcomes; symptom benefit lasts 9 to 12 months. Recent abstracts have shown promising results in idiopathic DO, but Botox is expensive. For review see Sahai et al.[24]

Intravesical Resiniferatoxin (RTX) Installation
This has been used for several years for neuropathic DO, with considerable success. This agent acts to desensitize the vanilloid receptors in the bladder lining, which normally convey the sense of urgency. Small clinical trials have also been undertaken in idiopathic DO, showing early promise. The solution is very cheap; results last about three months. For review see Cruz.[9]

CONCLUSIONS
Idiopathic detrusor overactivity is often very distressing for patients, because they cannot predict when they will leak. It is also rather frustrating for the clinician, because we do not yet understand the cause of the condition, and we have no "cure". Patients need to be treated as sympathetically as possible, with meticulous bladder training, and attempts to find the best therapy for each woman. It is also important to emphasize that a great deal of research is ongoing, to discover the cause and find better treatments.

References
1. Amarenco G, Ismael SS, Even-Scneider A, Raibaut P, Demaille-Wlodyka S, Parratte B, Derdraon J (2003) Urodynamic effect of acute transcutaneous posterior tibial nerve stimulation in overactive bladder. J Urol 169:2210–2215.
2. Awad SA, AlSahrani HM, Gajewski JB, Bourque-Kehoe AA (1998) Long-term results and complications of augmentation ileocystoplasty for idiopathic urge incontinence in women. Br J Urol 81: 569–573.
3. Benness C (1992) Vaginal oestradiol for postmenopausal urinary symptoms, a double blind placebo controlled study. Proceedings of FIGO, Stockholm.
4. Bosch J, Groen J (1995) Sacral (S3) segmental nerve stimulation as a treatment for urge incontinence in patients with detrusor instability: Results of chronic electrical stimulation using an implantable neural prosthesis. J Urol 154:504–509.
5. Bower WF, Moore KH, Adams R (1998) A urodynamic study of surface neuromodulation versus sham in detrusor instability and sensory urgency. J Urol 106:2133–2136.

6. Brubaker L, Benson JT, Bent A, Clark A, Shott S (1997) Transvaginal electrical stimulation for female urinary incontinence. Am J Obstet Gynecol 177:536–540.

7. Burton G (1994) A randomised cross over trial comparing oxybutnin taken three times a day or taken "when needed". Neurourol Urodyn 13:351–352.

8. Chang PL (1988) Urodynamic studies in acupuncture for women with frequency, urgency and dysuria. J Urol 140:563–566.

9. Cruz F (2002) Vanilloid receptor and detrusor instability. Urology 59 (Suppl 5A):51–60.

10. Delaere KP, Debruyne FM, Michiels H, Moonen W (1980) Prolonged bladder distension in the management of the unstable bladder. J Urol 124:334–336.

11. Freeman RM (1987) A psychological approach to detrusor instability incontinence in women. Stress Med 3:9–14.

12. Goldberg RP, Galloway NT, Sand PK (2004) Extracorporeal electromagnetic stimulation therapy. In: Bourcier AP, McGuire EJ, Abrams P (eds) Pelvic floor disorders. Elsevier Saunders, Philadelphia, Chapter 30, pp 291–296.

13. Govier FE, Litwiller S, Nitti V, Kreder KJ, Rosenblatt P (2001) Cutaneous afferent neuromodulation for the refractory overactive bladder: Results of a multicenter study. J Urol 165:1193–1198.

14. Hasan ST, Robson WA, Pridie AK, Neal DE (1994) Outcome of transcutaneous electrical stimulation in patients with detrusor instability. Neurourol Urodyn 13:349–350.

15. Hassouna MM (2003) Sacral nerves neurostimulation. In: Drutz HP, Herschorn S, Diamant NE (eds) Female pelvic medicine and reconstructive pelvic surgery. Springer, London, Chapter 27, pp 299–312.

16. Herbison P, Hay-Smith J, Ellis G, Moore KH (2003) Effectiveness of anticholinergic drugs compared with placebo in the treatment of overactive bladder: Systematic review. Br Med J 326:841–847.

17. Kumar V, Cross R, Chess-William R, Chapple C (2005) Recent advances in basic science for overactive bladder. Curr opin Urol 15: 222–226.

18. Leng WW, Blalock HJ, Fredriksson WH, English SF, McGuire EJ (1999) Enterocystoplasty or detrusor myectomy? Comparison of indications and outcomes for bladder augmentation. J Urol 161: 758–763.

19. Moore KH, Gilpin SA, Dixon JS, Richmond DH, Sutherst JR (1992) An increase of presumptive sensory nerves of the urinary bladder in idiopathic detrusor instability. Br J Urol 70:370–372.

20. Morris A, O'Sullivan R, Donkley P, Moore KH (2005) Extracorporeal magnetic stimulation in female detrusor overactivity simultaneous cystometry testing and a randomizedsham controlled trial. Neurorol and Urodyn (in press).

21. Morris AR, Westbrook JI, Moore KH (2003) Idiopathic detrusor over-activity in women—A 5–10 year longitudinal study of outcomes. Neurourol Urodyn 22:460–462.

22. Philp T, Shah PJR, Worth PHL (1988) Acupuncture in the treatment of bladder instability. Br J Urol 61:490–493.

23. Ramsden PS, Smith M, Dunn M, Ardran GM (1976) Distention therapy for the unstable bladder: Later results including an assessment of repeat distensions. Br J Urol 48:623–629.

24. Sahai A, Khan M, Fowler CJ, Dasgupta P (2005) Botulinum toxin for the treatment of lower urinary tract symptoms: A review. Neurourol Urodyn 24:2–12.

25. Scheepens WA, Van Koeveringe GA, DeBie RA, Weil EH, Van Kerrebroeck PE (2002) Long term efficacy and safety results of the two stage implantation techniques in sacral neuromodulation. Br J Urol Int 90:840–845.

26. Shaker HS, Hassouna MM (1998) Sacral nerve root neuromodulation: Effective treatment for refractory urge incontinence. J Urol 159:1516–1519.

27. Smet P, Moore KH, Jonavicius J (1997) Distribution and colocalisation of calcitonin gene-related peptide, tachykinins, and vasoactive intestinal peptide in normal and idiopathic unstable human urinary bladder. Lab Invest 77:37–49.

28. Swami KS, Feneley RC, Hammonds JC, Abrams P (1998) Detrusor myectomy for detrusor overactivity: A minimum 1 year followup. Br J Urol 81:68–72.

Chapter 8
Anal Incontinence and Disorders of Obstructive Defecation

Before moving on to surgical treatment of stress incontinence, or management of prolapse, we must briefly consider the disorders of defecation.

Many patients with urinary incontinence or prolapse have anal incontinence, recurrent straining with constipation, or other aspects of obstructive defecation. Because surgery may be considered for the defecation disorder, and in some pelvic floor units, these surgeries are performed simultaneously with bladder/prolapse procedures, such conditions are dealt with here.

BASIC PHYSIOLOGY OF ANAL CONTINENCE AND DEFECATION FOR THE GYNECOLOGIST

Because the anal continence mechanism and the physiology of defecation are not part of normal registrar training in gynecology, the doctor who works in a urogynecology unit needs a basic outline before the treatment of defecation disorders can be understood.

Anal continence depends upon the following.

1. Stool consistency (watery diarrhea alone can cause incontinence)
2. The ability of the rectum to distend up to normal volumes
3. The sensory input from the anal canal and rectum
4. The strength and innervation of the internal and external anal sphincters

The first problem is unique to the bowel (although infected urine can cause bladder incontinence). The second and third problems are rather like those seen in an overactive bladder, where the bladder wall may be noncompliant, and the subepithelial nerves are dysfunctional. The fourth problem is rather like that of stress incontinence (weak sphincters), except that the anal sphincters are more complex.

Several theories exist as to the mechanism of anal continence. In the 1970s the main theory was that the normal puborectalis muscle caused an acute anorectal angle, so that during rises in intra-abdominal pressure, the rectum was forced down upon the anal canal, with a "kink" at the puborectalis muscle, so that feces were denied access to the anal canal. Arising from this concept, the operation of post-anal repair was developed, to restore the anorectal angle and improve continence. This operation is still performed today, although success rates are very variable (see below).

Later studies showed that continence was really dependent upon the sphincters and the puborectalis muscle acting together. When the pressure in the rectum rises, the contractility of the anal sphincters increases, by neurological mechanisms. Thus operations to repair the anal sphincter, which do not increase the anorectal angle, also improve continence.

Even later, it was realized that continence also depends on awareness of rectal filling. This gives one the ability to distinguish whether the rectal contents are gas (when they could be passed in a private location, not necessarily a toilet), or feces, in which case the external sphincter can be contracted voluntarily while looking for a toilet. The anal canal is highly able to discriminate light touch, pain, and temperature. In contrast, the rectum is not very sensitive to these impulses. Instead, rectal sensation is conveyed by stretch receptors within the pelvic floor muscles, that respond to the bulk phenomenon of rectal distension.

Distension of the rectum (by feces or flatus) causes relaxation of the internal anal sphincter, along with contraction of the external anal sphincter. This allows the contents of the rectum to enter the sensitive anal canal (but prevents escape of the contents from the anus). Once the contents enter the anal canal, the nerves sense whether gas or feces are present. This is called the anal sampling reflex.

The sensitivity of the anal mucosa declines with age and menopause, partly explaining the increasing prevalence of anal incontinence in older women. Obviously there is no surgical cure for denervation/declining sensitivity of the anal mucosa.

Filling of the rectum is normally first sensed at volumes of 10–70 ml. Maximum capacity is about 300 ml. Rectal distension initiates contractions of smooth muscle in the rectal wall, which cause the desire to defecate at "fullness". This normal compliance of the rectal wall is reduced after pelvic irradiation, with inflammatory bowel disease, and sometimes after denervation following radical pelvic surgery.

Finally, strength and innervation of the sphincters are a vital component of continence. The Internal Anal Sphincter (IAS) is continuous with the circular muscle in the wall of the rectum (see Figure 8.1). It is in a constant state of tonic contraction, to promote continence. This provides the so-called "high-pressure zone" in the resting state, about 2 cm from the anal verge.

The high-pressure zone also receives a 15% contribution from the three "anal cushions" that have a rich arterial supply, and behave like erectile tissue. They are engorged with blood when the IAS is relaxed, and form a seal. Their pressure is higher in those with hemorrhoids, and can be damaged by vigorous hemorrhoidectomy. Inadvertent division, or marked thinning, of the IAS (ie after some vaginal deliveries) is associated with fecal soiling in up to 40% of cases.

The External Anal Sphincter (EAS) is continuous with the puborectalis muscle (see Figure 8.2). Although the EAS is stri-

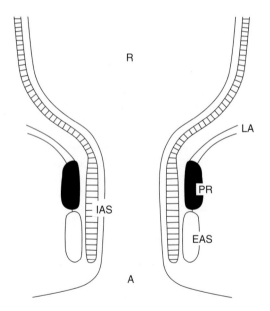

FIGURE 8.1. Anterior–posterior view of anorectal musculature: R, rectum; A, analcanal; IAS, internal anal sphincter; EAS, external anal sphincter; PR, puborectalis; LA, levator ani. (Reprinted with permission from Swash M (2002) Electrophysiological investigation of the posterior pelvic floor musculature. In: Pemberton JH, Swash M, Henry MM, (eds) The pelvic floor: Its function and disorders, WB Saunders p 214; Copyright 2002, Elsevier.)

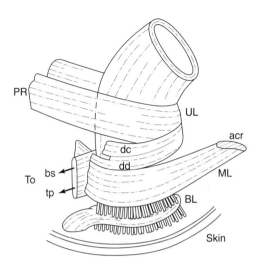

FIGURE 8.2. Lateral view of anorectal muscles. PR, puborectalis; UL, upper loop; DC, decussating fibers of puborectalis that blend with the longitudinal muscle of the rectum; DD, decussating fibers that join the perineal body; ML, middle loop; ACR, anococcygeal raphe; BS, bulbospongiosus; TP, deep transverse perinei; BL, basal loop, perforated by fibers of the conjoint longitudinal layer. (Reprinted with permission from Bogduk N. (1996) Issues in anatomy: The external anal sphincter revised. Aust N Z J Surg 66(9):626–629, Blackwell Publishing.)

ated muscle, and is under voluntary control, it is also in a constant state of contraction to promote continence. During cough, the EAS tightens reflexively. Ultrasound studies of the EAS have shown that about 35% of women delivered by forceps have a partial or complete laceration of the EAS, which generally does not recover and also contributes to anal incontinence.

The motor innervation to the EAS is via the pudendal nerve. Prolonged bearing down in the second stage of labor is associated with a traction neurapraxia of the pudendal nerve, which may not recover. This partly explains the association between prolonged second stage and anal incontinence.

If rectal sensation is poor, and rectal compliance is reduced, and if the sphincters are also weak, then patients can experience anal incontinence before they even get the desire to defecate.

The Act of Defecation

The defecation mechanism is still not completely understood, despite extensive research.

■ Stool comes down from the sigmoid colon to the rectum, by peristalsis.

■ Stretch receptors in the pelvic floor detect the stool in the rectum, giving the urge to defecate.

■ The anal sampling reflex (internal sphincter relaxes, external sphincter stays closed) occurs; the anal mucosa senses whether stool or gas is present and conveys this to the brain.

■ If defecation is not socially convenient, the pelvic floor muscles and the puborectalis contract. This propels feces back up into the sigmoid colon and the internal sphincter contracts again.

■ Once the toilet is reached, the pelvic floor muscles are relaxed while sitting on the toilet, allowing the perineum to descend.

■ Both sphincters are relaxed. Puborectalis opens.

■ The patient gives a Valsalva maneuver to raise intra-abdominal pressure.

■ The bolus of feces is expelled. Upon completion, a closing reflex tightens the external sphincter.

OVERVIEW OF ANAL INCONTINENCE
Anal incontinence is really "the last taboo." Patients are deeply ashamed if they soil themselves, and usually consider it far worse than urinary incontinence. Questions must be phrased very tactfully; eg, do you ever lose bowel material on your underwear?

Anal incontinence is actually not uncommon. Large prevalence studies of community-dwelling women indicate that about 2–14% of women have anal incontinence, with up to 47% of those in nursing homes.[6] As can be seen from the discussion of the physiology of defecation, the pathophysiology of anal incontinence is often multifactorial. Full details of assessment of such patients are available in the text by Pemberton et al.[7] The history assessment is described in Chapter 1. The Wexner score should be used to measure severity of anal incontinence (shown in Chapter 5). Considerable detail about previous colorectal surgery, previous radiation, inflammatory bowel disease, and so on is needed. Physical examination requires greater attention to anal sphincter tone, perineal descent, pelvic innervation, and the like.

We encourage any patient with regular fecal incontinence to be fully assessed by a dedicated colorectal surgeon. Such a surgeon is part of our Unit, so that case notes and nursing staff are shared. On the other hand, patients with minor incontinence to flatus or rare incontinence to liquid stool may benefit from conservative pelvic floor muscle training.[4]

The common tests of anorectal function for patients with anal incontinence comprise the following.

Anorectal manometry tests the magnitude of the resting anal pressure at the high-pressure zone (85% comes from IAS rhythmic slow wave contractions, 15% from tonic contraction of EAS). The most common method is a water-perfused catheter containing four recording channels, to detect pressure at various points along the rectum/anal canal, with a balloon at the end. After testing baseline resting pressures, the patient is asked to cough (pressures should rise briefly, to prevent incontinence) then to squeeze the EAS, which gives the voluntary "squeeze pressure". The rectal balloon is then distended with fluid to elicit a brief drop in anal pressure, showing competency of the "sampling reflex".

Pudendal nerve conduction studies test the innervation of the sphincters, by measuring whether the time taken to conduct a stimulus is delayed (the conduction latency). A stimulating electrode, mounted on a gloved finger, is inserted into the rectum; the fingertip is placed on the ischial spine (near the pudendal nerve), with a recording electrode at the external anal sphincter. The latency is the time taken for the electrical stimulus to reach the recording electrode. The test requires an experienced person to produce reliable measurements and thus some Units have discarded it, although it was a standard test for many years. Allen et al[1] used this test to provide the first evidence of intra-partum damage to the pudendal nerve, although long-term followup showed that most patients' nerve conduction recovered over time. Prolonged straining at stool is also associated with prolonged pudendal nerve conduction times.

Single fiber electromyography is another way of detecting nerve damage. Because denervation of a skeletal muscle is accompanied by re-innervation from neighboring axons, a single fiber EMG electrode can detect multiple axons firing within a small area of the muscle, to indicate that it has been damaged, then re-innervation has occurred.

Anal mucosal sensitivity testing tests the adequacy of anal sensation (that is needed for the anorectal sampling reflex). A ring electrode mounted on a Foley catheter is placed in the anal canal. A tiny current (up to 0.1 milliamperes) is delivered: the patient states when she can feel a tingling sensation. Standard normal values have been derived.

Endo-Anal Ultrasound is now the best way to measure whether the sphincters are intact, using a rotating probe or a linear probe. Defects of the EAS are detected very accurately. This technique was used by Sultan et al[9] to show that about 35%

of parous women have defects of the EAS. This does not necessarily mean that they will respond to surgery.

TREATMENT OF ANAL INCONTINENCE

Management involves a large range of conservative and surgical treatments. A short summary is provided; for details see Eccersly and William.[3]

Pelvic floor muscle training to teach the patient to contract the external anal sphincter, similar to that in urinary incontinence. Biofeedback is often used, by a rectal EMG sensing device, to enhance patients' awareness of their ability to contract. Electrical stimulation of the muscle has also been used (as for stress incontinence). Success ranges from 12% to 90% cure/major benefit for anal incontinence.[4]

Regulation of diet to avoid watery stool is often successful for patients who only leak when they have liquid feces. Also 2–3 dessert spoons of Metamucil or psyllium husks are dissolved in a small amount of water (100–150 ml) to thicken the stool.

The drug Imodium (Loperamide) is also used to thicken the stool; it also increases the resting tone of the anal sphincters to promote continence.

Anal sphincter repair (sphincteroplasty) involves dissecting the damaged ends of the external sphincter, freeing them up enough to be laid across each other and sutured, in an "overlap repair". When performed for obstetric lacerations of the sphincter, continence is achieved in about 80%. Success is best when the pudendal nerve to the sphincter is intact. Repairing the internal sphincter does <u>not</u> improve success.

Post-anal repair involves plication of the puborectalis muscle posterior to the anorectal junction. The posterior aspect of the external sphincter is usually reinforced with sutures as well. The operation is designed to increase the anorectal angle (originally thought to be very important to the continence mechanism). Audit in the mid-1990s showed that less than 50% of patients have improved continence at two years, so the procedure is less commonly performed now.

The dynamic graciloplasty procedure involves taking a segment of gracilis muscle from the inner aspect of the thigh, then tunneling it under the pubic bone to wrap it around the anal sphincter. Because the gracilis is mainly a "fast twitch" Type II muscle that cannot maintain a contraction over time, an implanted electrical stimulator is applied to the muscle, to convert it to a slow-twitch postural-type muscle over six months. The patient uses a control device to turn off the stimulus in order to defecate. Data from 1999 indicates 66% success rate.[3]

OVERVIEW OF THE DISORDERS OF OBSTRUCTIVE DEFECATION

In the urogynecology patient, the main problems comprise constipation, incomplete evacuation with a need to digitate the vagina, and post-defecation soiling. These symptoms often coexist with rectocele, but such patients are often referred to the colorectal surgeon rather than the urogynecologist.

Debate exists about who should manage rectocele. In our Unit, such patients are often assessed jointly by the urogynecology team and the colorectal team, then a decision is made as to who should manage the patient. The colorectal perspective is given here, derived from experience in our Unit.

Constipation

When patients complain of constipation, only about a third of them are actually concerned about infrequent defecation; the rest are worried about straining at stool, or passing hard stools.

The definition of constipation has recently been standardized, now called the "Rome definition", as a patient who has two or more of the following, for at least 12 months, when not taking laxatives.[2]

■ Straining during >25% of bowel movements (BM)
■ Sensation of incomplete evacuation in >25% of BM
■ Hard or pellety stools on >25% of BM
■ Less than three stools passed per week

It is useful to employ the Bristol stool chart to define what type of stool the patient passes (Figure 8.3).

Other symptoms such as need to digitate to defecate, abdominal cramps, bloating, and so on do not feature in the Rome definition but help one to assess the severity of the constipation. Depending upon the definition used, constipation affects about 4% of the population, but about 17% of those aged 30–64, and 40% of those over age 65. It is common in urogynecological patients.

Assessing the Causes of Constipation

Before one treats constipation, one must seek nonbowel (secondary) causes. Some can be reversed. Others indicate that management may be difficult. These include:

THE BRISTOL STOOL FORM SCALE

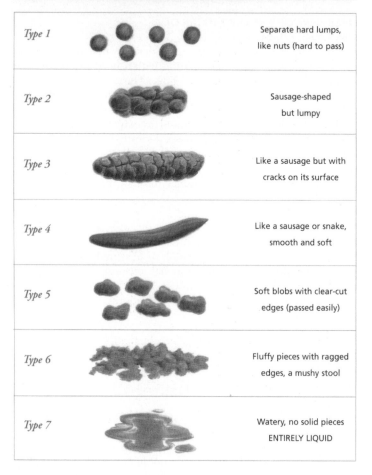

Type 1		Separate hard lumps, like nuts (hard to pass)
Type 2		Sausage-shaped but lumpy
Type 3		Like a sausage but with cracks on its surface
Type 4		Like a sausage or snake, smooth and soft
Type 5		Soft blobs with clear-cut edges (passed easily)
Type 6		Fluffy pieces with ragged edges, a mushy stool
Type 7		Watery, no solid pieces ENTIRELY LIQUID

FIGURE 8.3. The Bristol Stool Chart. (Reprinted by kind permission of Dr. K. W. Heaton, Reader in Medicine at the University of Bristol, Copyright 2000 Norgine Ltd.)

- Endocrine causes; hypothyroidism, hypercalcaemia, diabetic autonomic neuropathy
- Neurological disorders; Parkinson's disease, multiple sclerosis, autonomic neuropathy

- Psychiatric causes: depression, anorexia, sexual abuse
- Narcotic analgesic drugs
- Cardiac drugs (nifedipine, verapamil, disopyramide, amiodarone, flecainide)
- Antidepressants (clomipramine, fluoxetine, venlafaxine, sertraline, paroxetine)
- Tranquilizers (alpraxolam, olanzapine, risperidone)
- Lipid-lowering drugs (lovastatin, pravachol, cholestyramine)
- Miscellaneous drugs; bromocriptine, valproic acid, ondansetron

Once secondary causes are excluded, other bowel disorders that can manifest as constipation should be considered, such as diverticulosis, polyps, stricture, ischemia/bowel obstruction, and malignancy. One is left with four main types of constipation.

Simple constipation describes patients who have a mild to moderate degree of difficult or infrequent passage of stool, which responds quickly to increased fluid/fiber intake.

Constipation—predominant irritable bowel syndrome includes such patients mainly complaining of abdominal pain, who are commonly young women, and is not considered further here.

Idiopathic slow transit constipation is a rare disorder, generally affecting young to middle-aged women who seldom feel the urge to defecate and have a very poor response to laxatives or bulking agents.

Outlet obstruction/evacuation disorders comprise:

Rectal mucosal prolapse is a surgical problem, not considered further here.

Intussusception is a prolapse of the anorectal mucosa down into the anal canal; the functional significance of this radiological finding is controversial.

Anismus is a condition in which patients have trouble emptying the rectum because they experience involuntary spasm of the striated pelvic floor muscles or of the puborectalis muscle (see below, under biofeedback therapy).

Rectocele is a prolapse of the anterior wall of the rectum into the vagina.

The basic investigations that are used to distinguish these four types of primary constipation are as follows.

Anorectal manometry studies (as per fecal incontinence) but with the addition of a balloon expulsion test to elicit spasm of the striated muscles seen in anismus.

A *colonic transit study* involves the ingestion of radio-opaque markers over three days; then an abdominal X-ray is taken on day 4 (or later if markers still present). In normal patients, the gut transit time is 36 hours so all markers should be expelled by day 4; a prolonged test suggests idiopathic slow transit constipation.

A *defecating proctogram* (Figure 8.4) is an X-ray test of the act of defecating a radio-opaque porridgelike mixture. It identifies the site and size of rectocele (as well as other defects). If contrast material is trapped in the rectocele after defecation, this can also lead to post-defecation soiling (as the feces slowly seeps out from the pocket).

Colorectal surgeons classify rectocele as low, middle, and high. Middle and high defects are more likely to be associated with enterocele, and thus referred for gynecological repair. A low rectocele is more likely to be associated with scarring and shortening of the perineal body and anal sphincter; thus colorectal surgeons commonly repair these defects.

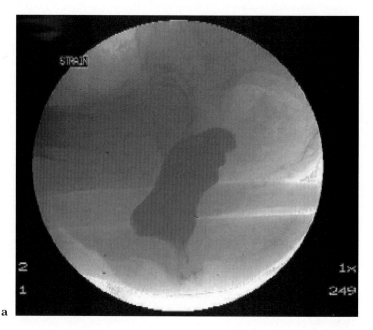

a

FIGURE 8.4. Defecating proctogram. **(a)** The bulging of the rectocele anteriorly into the vagina.

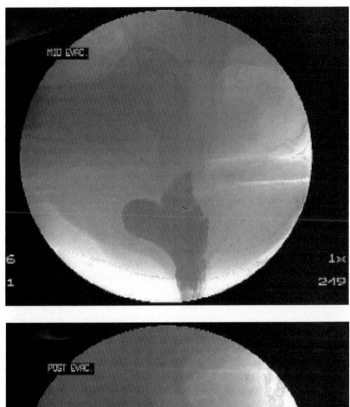

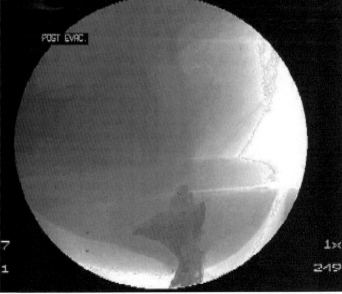

FIGURE 8.4. **(b)** Defecation, with "hold-up" in the rectocele. **(c)** Post-defecation film, with contrast trapped in the anterior rectocele.

OVERVIEW OF TREATMENT OF DISORDERS OF DEFECATION

Simple constipation is treated as discussed in Chapter Two. A dedicated nurse continence advisor or continence physiotherapist can also help such patients to:

Learn the correct position for defecation (feet elevated to accentuate relaxation of the anorectal angle).

Modify their lifestyle so they have enough time to relax and defecate properly as soon as they have the call to stool. Postponement of the defecation impulse because of a busy schedule is a major factor in constipated individuals.

Constipation—predominate IBS is difficult to treat (not within the remit of this chapter).

Idiopathic slow transit constipation, once suspected on the basic tests, requires a more complex study of colonic motility to elicit a reduction in myoelectrical activity, as well as serious effort with laxative therapy. If this fails, surgical removal of the colon with ileorectal anastomosis may be indicated, although diarrhea may result.

Anismus is treated by biofeedback. Similar intra-rectal EMG devices are used to help patients to relax their anal spincters and puborectalis during the act of defecation.

Rectocele may be treated by transrectal repair; see Figure 8.5. The advantage of the colorectal approach is that any associated anal sphincter defect can be repaired at the same time as the trans-anal repair. However, if the anal sphincter is intact, controversy exists about trans-anal repair because this approach requires the use of anal retractors, which may stretch the sphincters. Anal incontinence after trans-anal repair of rectocele can occur in up to 30% of patients, although 92–97% of patients will have complete resolution of the hernia defect, with resolution of the need to digitate in order to evacuate.

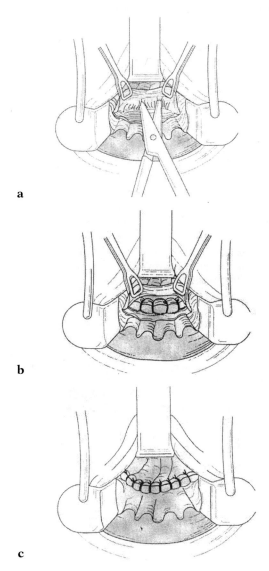

a

b

c

FIGURE 8.5. Trans-anal repair of rectocele. **(a)** A mucosal flap is raised around the anterior half of the anal canal. **(b)** The anterior rectal wall muscle is folded down to the distal anal canal and imbricated, so as to abolish the rectocele sac. **(c)** The now redundant mucosa is excised; the new muco-cutaneon function is restored across the anterior lumen of the anal canal. (Reprinted with permission from Lawler LP, Fleshman JW (2002) Solitary rectal ulcer, rectocele, hemorrhoids and pelvic pain. In: Pemberton JH, Swash M, Henry MM (eds) The pelvic floor: its function and disorders. WB Saunders, p 368. Copyright 2002, Elsevier.)

CONCLUSIONS

Anal incontinence and disorders of defecation are more common than is generally appreciated. Such problems need to be elicited carefully in urogynecololgy patients. If minor and rare, conservative therapy may help, but if the problem gives rise to major symptoms, full investigation is needed. Treatment may be carried out in conjuction with the urogynecological condition in certain cases.

A Note Regarding Obstetric Trauma as a Cause of Anal Incontinence

In the last 15 years, colorectal surgeons and obstetricians have become increasingly aware that the management of the second stage of labor has tremendous impact upon the likelihood of anal incontinence developing during a woman's life.

This subject is vast and controversial. It cannot be adequately dealt with in a short practical text. This does not mean it is not important.

The following is a list of some landmark papers that give an overview of the subject.

Engel AF, Kamm MA, Sultan AH, Bartram CI, Nicholls RJ (1994) Anterior anal sphincter repair in patients with obstetric trauma. Br J Surg 81:1231–124.

Fitzpatrick M, Behan M, O'Connell R, O'Herlihy C (2000) A randomized clinical trial comparing primary overlap with approximation repair of third-degree obstetric tears. Am J Obstet Gynecol 183:1220–1224.

Kamm MA (1998) Faecal incontinence: Clinical review. BMJ 316:528–532.

Kammerer-Doak DN, Wesol AB, Rogers RG, Dominguez, Dorin MH (1999) A prospective cohort study of women after primary repair of obstetric anal sphincter laceration. Am J Obstet Gynecol 181:1317–1323.

MacArthur C, Bick DE, Keighley MRB (1997) Faecal incontinence after childbirth. Br J Obstet Gynaecol 104:46–50.

MacArthur C, Glazener CM, Wilson PD, Herbison GP, Gee H, Lang GD, et al. (2001) Obstetric practice and faecal incontinence three months after delivery. BJOG 108:678–683.

Malouf A, Norton C, Engel AF, Nicholls RJ, Kamm MA (2000) Long-term results of anterior overlapping anal-sphincter repair for obstetric trauma. Lancet 355:260–265.

Norton C, Hosker G, Brazzelli M, Behan M, Walsh D, O'Connell PR (2000) Biofeedback and/or sphincter exercises for the treatment of faecal incontinence in adults. Cochrane Database Syst Rev CD 002111.

Reiger NA, Wattchow DA, Sarre RG, Cooper SJ, Rich CA, Saccone GT, et al. (1997) Prospective trial of pelvic floor retraining in patients with faecal incontinence. Dis Colon Rectum 40:821–826.

Royal College of Obstetricians and Gynaecologists (2001) Management of third and fourth degree perineal tears following vaginal delivery. RCOG Guideline No.29. London: RCOG Press. Available from RCOG Web site.

Spence-Jones C, Kamm MA, Henry MM, Hudson CN (1997) Bowel dysfunction: A pathogenic factor in uterovaginal prolapse and urinary stress incontinence. Br J Obstet Gynaecol 104:311–315.

Sultan AH, Kamm MA (1997) Faecal incontinence after childbirth. Br J Obstet Gynaecol 104:979–982.

Sultan AH, Kamm MA, Hudson CN (1995) Obstetric perineal tears: an audit of training. J Obstet Gynaecol 15:19–23.

Sultan AH, Kamm MA, Hudson CN, Bartram CI (1994) Third degree obstetric anal sphincter tears: Risk factors & outcome of primary repair. BMJ 308:887–891.

Sultan AH, Kamm MA, Hudson CN, Thomas JM, Bartram CI (1993) Anal sphincter disruption during vaginal delivery. N Engl J Med 329: 1905–1911.

Swash M (1993) Faecal incontinence: Childbirth is responsible for most cases. BMJ 307:636–637.

Wood J, Amos L, Reiger N (1998) Third degree anal sphincter tears: Risk factors and outcome. Aust N Z J Obstet Gynaecol 38:414–417.

References

1. Allen RE, Hosker GL, Smith AR, Warrell DW (1990) Pelvic floor damage and childbirth, a neurophysiological study. Br J Obstet Gynaecology 97:770–779.

2. Drossman DA, Thompson WG, Talley NJ, et al (1990) Identification of sub-groups of functional gastrointestinal disorders. Gastroenterol Int 3:159–172.

3. Eccersley AJ, William NS (2002) Fecal incontinence—Pathophysiology and management. In: Pemberton JH, Swash M, Henry MM (eds) The pelvic floor, its function and disorders. WB Saunders, London, Chapter 24, pp 341–357.

4. Enck P, Frauke M (2002) Biofeedback in pelvic floor disorders. In: Pemberton JH, Swash M, Henry MM (eds) The pelvic floor, its function and disorders. WB Saunders, London, Chapter 27, p 393–404.

5. Fynes M, Marshall K, et al (1999) A prospective randomized study comparing the effect of augmented biofeedback with sensory biofeedback alone on fecal incontinence after obstetric trauma. Dis Colon Rectum 42:753–761.

6. Norton C, Christiansen J, Butler U, et al (2001) Anal incontinence. In: Abrams P, Cardozo L, Khoury S, Wein A (eds): 2nd International Consultation on Incontinence. WHO. Plymouth, Plymbridge, pp 985–1043.

7. Pemberton JH, Swash M, Henry MM (eds) (2002) The pelvic floor, its function and disorders. WB Saunders, London, pp 172–213.
8. Reiger N, Wattchow D, et al (1997) Prospective trial of pelvic floor retraining in patients with fecal incontinence. Dis Colon Rectum 40:821–826.
9. Sultan AH, Kamm MA, Hudson CN, Thomas JM, Bartram CI (1993) Anal-sphincter disruption during vaginal delivery. N Engl J Med 329:1905–1911.

Chapter 9
Surgery for Urodynamic Stress Incontinence

INTRODUCTION

Prior to the late 1960s, patients who leaked when they coughed usually underwent an anterior colporrhaphy (anterior repair) with a bladder neck buttress. Urodynamic testing was not commonplace until the late 1970s.

Once urodynamic studies were introduced, it was realized that coughing can provoke a detrusor contraction. Thus many women who underwent anterior repair did not obtain cure (because they had an element of detrusor overactivity). This poor success rate was one of the reasons that gynecologists became interested in performing urodynamics tests (to improve their surgical cure rates), and was one stimulus to the establishment of urogynecology as a subspecialty.

BLADDER NECK BUTTRESS

This procedure is still used in highly selected cases. For example, if a woman mainly complains of prolapse due to cystocele, but is found to have a minor element of stress incontinence on urodynamic testing, then it may be reasonable to perform this procedure. This is particularly true if an elderly woman with prolapse and stress incontinence is found to have an underactive detrusor at urodynamics; one may counsel her that a simple repair with buttress for her stress incontinence is not likely to cause voiding difficulty. The evidence for this comes from retrospective case series, rather than randomized controlled trial.[10]

The bladder neck buttress involves the following (see Figure 9.1).

- Insert urethral catheter with 5 ml balloon (to delineate urethrovesical junction).
- Inject local anesthetic with adrenaline into subcutaneous plane.

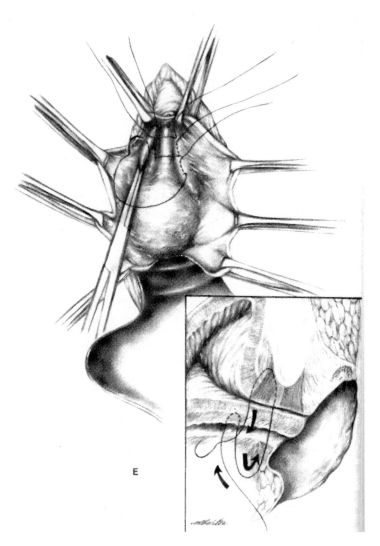

FIGURE 9.1. Bladder neck buttress procedure. The sutures pass deeply through the periurethral endopelvic fascia on the posterior aspect of the symphysis pubis (arrow). (Reprinted with permission from Thompson JD, Rock JA (eds) (1992) Te Linde's operative gynecology, 7 edn. Lippincott Williams & Wilkins, Philadelphia.

■ Dissect vaginal epithelium off the bladder and proximal urethra.
■ Use a small needle with 1 Vicryl or nonabsorbable suture.
■ Place three mattress sutures at the bladder neck and proximal urethra to plicate (or buttress) the periurethral fascia that borders the levator hiatus.

The goal is to assist closure of an open bladder neck, but if done correctly it will also elevate the urethrovesical junction in the retropubic space. This procedure was first described by Kelly in 1913, who reported an initial subjective success rate of 90%, but this decreased to 60% subjectively continent over five years.

For further details of associated anterior repair for cystocele, see Chapter 10 (prolapse). For post-operative management of voiding function, see Colposuspension below.

COLPOSUSPENSION

From about 1970 until the late 1990s, the most common procedure for USI was the colposuspension. This is still a very useful procedure if the patient requires an abdominal procedure for some other reason.

The procedure is mainly indicated for USI in the presence of urethral hypermobility. If previous surgery has created a fixed, nonmobile urethra, consideration should be given to performing an abdomino-vaginal sling or injecting collagen (but see discussion of TVT). The colposuspension is also highly effective in correcting cystocele.

Pre-Operative Consent Discussion

Before consenting a patient for colposuspension, ensure that she understands fully the 5–15% risk of developing de novo detrusor overactivity. Patients can be very distressed if they have an operation because they leak when they play tennis, but afterwards have to void frequently and leak with unpredictable urge, not to mention nocturia. Such angry patients are commonly referred to a tertiary urogynecology unit!

Also, ensure that the patient understands the 2–5% risk of longer term voiding dysfunction (with approximately 0.5% risk of clean intermittent self-catheterization, CISC). Some urogynecologists ask the patient to meet with a nurse continence advisor to explain CISC before carrying out the operation.

Post-Operative Convalescence

This is similar to abdominal hysterectomy, eg the first week at home should be spent in quiet leisure (reading books, watching

TV, etc). The next five weeks are "light duties" (including driving locally, ordinary shopping, with regular rest periods). At six weeks, normal activity resumes (including intercourse, swimming, light gym exercise), but with no heavy lifting for a further six weeks.

Patients want to know the chance of failure. Objective success rates depend very much on the outcome measure chosen. The original series by Burch[3] revealed a cure rate of 93% ($n = 143$) at approximately 2 years, as judged by a stress test at 250 ml and a lateral X-ray with a metal bead chain in the urethra (to look for stress leak or an open bladder neck). The cure rate at a mean of 14 years followup (range 10–20 years, $n = 109$) was 80% on one-hour pad testing.[1]

The Technique of Colposuspension
This involves the following. See Figure 9.2.

- Place a 14–16 gauge catheter (easy to feel vaginally) in the urethra.
- Inflate 5-ml balloon (30-ml balloon is too big, will get in the way).
- Make a Pfannenstiel incision.
- Access the retropubic space (the Cave of Retzius).
- By careful dissection (to avoid large veins in this region), expose the back of the pubic bone and the lateral aspects of the urethra.
- The right-handed operator double gloves, and places the left hand in the vagina.
- With fingers on either side of the catheter in the vagina, define the urethrovesical junction (at the balloon).
- Place three Ethibond J-shaped sutures on either side of the urethrovesical junction.
- Attach each suture to the iliopectineal ligament at the back of the pubic bone.
- With the surgeon's left hand lifting up the vagina, the assistant ties the sutures onto the iliopectineal ligament.
- The surgeon dictates the degree of tension so as not to over-correct (tissue should not be taut, just comfortably elevated).
- Insert a drain to the retropubic space.
- Insert suprapubic catheter, empty the bladder, no vaginal pack.

Immediate Complications of Colposuspension
- Hemorrhage into the retropubic space, with a transfusion risk of about 0.5%

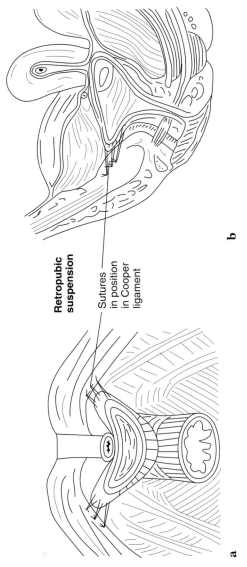

FIGURE 9.2. Colposuspension procedure. Three permanent sutures are placed through the endopelvic fascia (**a**) and passed through the iliopectineal ligament of Cooper (**b**).

■ Trauma to the bladder (inadvertent cystotomy) requiring repair and subsequent urethral catheter for 7–10 days, approximately 2–3%

Long-Term Complications of Colposuspension
■ Enterocele or rectocele 7–17% (but 25% at 14 years[1])
■ Dyspareunia 4%, because of acute retropubic angle of the anterior vaginal wall
■ Detrusor overactivity 5–15% (but note 22% incidence in Langer et al[9])
■ Recurrent bacterial cystitis 1–2% (but 5% at 12 years, Langer et al[9] and at 14 years[1])
■ Voiding difficulty 2–5%

Post-Operative Management for Colposuspension
■ Free drainage of SPC for 36–48 hours; patient unlikely to void due to pain of incision over this timeframe.
■ Commence trial of void at approximately 36 hours, if patient ambulant.
■ Once residual volumes less than 100 ml on three consecutive occasions, usually by day 5 postop, remove suprapubic catheter.

Double Voiding Technique
■ If residuals gradually getting lower but still not <100 ml at day 4–5,
■ Teach patient to
   —Void the first time in normal position.
   —Stand up, rotate the pelvis a few times to stimulate the afferent nerves.
   —Sit down, lean forward with elbows on knees.
   —"Drop" or purposefully relax, the pelvic floor muscles.
   —Remain so for two to three minutes, perhaps read a magazine, await further flow.

This often will produce another 50–100 ml, sufficient to give residual <100.

How to Manage Short-Term Voiding Difficulty
Note that the literature often does not define what is meant by "voiding difficulty". In this text, "short-term voiding difficulty" means the management of a temporary supra-pubic catheter (SPC), or self-catheterization, for up to four weeks. "Long-term voiding dysfunction" means that the temporary SPC required

removal, and thus CISC was instigated, from four weeks to permanently.

■ If patient is not voiding to completion by fifth postoperative day, and
  —Not suffering from persistent wound pain (hematoma/infection).
  —Able to defecate fully (no impacted feces or perineal pain from other repair).
  —Urine is not infected.
  —Double-emptying technique is being used.
  —But otherwise well and ready to plan discharge from hospital.
■ Discard the drainage bag.
■ Attach a Staubli valve or Flip Flow valve (Figure 9.3) to the SPC.
■ Teach patient to record own voided volumes and residual volumes on chart.
■ After training for 12 to 24 hours, using a "witches' hat" graduated collecting device placed in the toilet (Figure 9.3).
■ Send her home for three or four days to continue trial of void in home toilet.

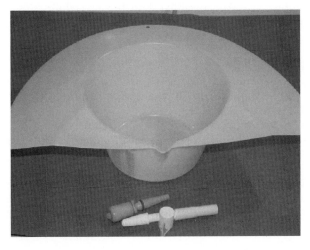

FIGURE 9.3. Witches' hat urine collection device and Staubi/Flip Flow valves.

■ Review back in clinic in three or four days with her residual volume chart.
■ Majority of patients will void well with this method.

How to Manage Long-Term Voiding Dysfunction

■ If unable to void after two–three weeks of home trial of void,
—The SPC site will become inflamed and painful.
■ If patient is almost voiding normally, Flucloxacillin 500 mg tds may help to preserve the SPC for a few more days.
■ After this, patient should be trained in Clean Intermittent Self-Catheterization (CISC), by a specialist nurse continence advisor because the SPC site will become inflamed.
■ Followup with a voided volume and residual chart, kept for 24 hours prior to each visit; should be every two weeks thereafter. If the bladder is kept well emptied by CISC, spontaneous resolution of the voiding dysfunction often occurs over three months.
■ Bad prognostic features are
—Patients with previous pelvic radiotherapy.
—Patients taking psychotropic drugs with anticholinergic properties.
—Patients who have undergone radical bowel resection with denervation of pelvic nerves.

THE ABDOMINO-VAGINAL SLING

Also known as the pubovaginal sling, this procedure is the time-honored operation for patients with previous failed continence surgery, particularly if:

■ There is persistent hypermobility on vaginal examination and videourodynamics (VCU).
■ If the urethra is fixed in the retropubic space (on VE and VCU), but
—The urethra closure pressure is low (below 20 cm).
—Or the Valsalva leak point pressure is low (below 60 cm).
—Then the abdomino-vaginal sling is worthwhile.

Note that if the urethra is fixed in the retropubic space but the urethral closure pressure or Valsalva leak point pressure is normal, then collagen/macroplastique injections may be worthwhile; see later section this chapter.

Pre-Operative Consent Discussion

This discussion is similar to that for the colposuspension, except that risk of voiding difficulty/dysfunction is probably higher, mean of 12.5% (range 3–32%); risk of de novo detrusor over-activity is similar (mean risk 10%, range 4–18%). The objective success rate after previous failed procedures is 86% (all data from Jarvis[10]).

After a procedure involving a Pfannenstiel incision and a vaginal incision, the first "quiet" week of the convalescence period should probably increase to two weeks, but light duties should still be appropriate at six weeks.

The abdomino-vaginal sling procedure entails the following (see Figure 9.4).

■ Insert 16 G Foley catheter into bladder with 5 ml balloon.
■ Make a wide Pfannenstiel incision.
■ Harvest a strip of rectus abdominus fascia 13 cm × 2 cm; wrap in moist gauze.
■ Dissect down to the retropubic space as for a colposuspension.
■ From below, incise the anterior vaginal wall as for an anterior repair, but should only need to dissect about 3 cm below the urethrovesical junction.
■ Working on a flat sterile surface, insert nylon 1.0 sutures to the four corners of the rectus sheath strip.
■ Insert a long narrow Bosman's packing forcep downwards from the retropubic space into the vagina, emerging at the urethrovesical junction (guided by the balloon of the catheter).
■ Bring the nylon sutures attached to the strip of sheath up into the abdominal wound (first on the left, then on the right).
■ Place the fascia strip under the urethrovesical junction.
■ Apply 2.0 Vicryl tacking sutures to the fascia at the edges of the vaginal wound to maintain the position of the strip at the urethrovesical junction.
■ Lift the nylon sutures into the abdominal wound, so as to place the fascial strip just under the urethra, with absolutely no tension.
■ Tie the nylon sutures at the four corners of the strip to the rectus abdominus fascia.
■ Close the abdominal and vaginal wounds in the traditional fashion.
■ Insert SPC. Insert drain to the retropubic space. Pack not mandatory.

Post-operative management is as for a colposuspension. Some surgeons perform this sling procedure using artificial mesh, but many prefer to harvest the patient's own (autologous)

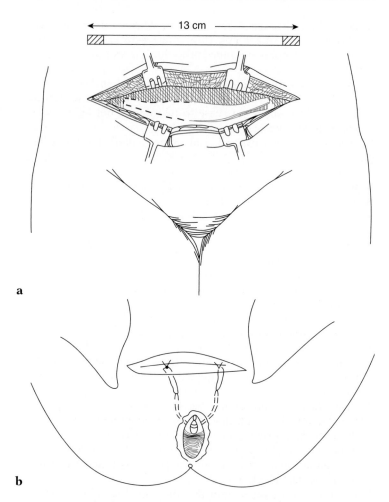

FIGURE 9.4. (**a**) Harvesting a strip of rectus abdominus fascia 13 × 2.5 cm. (**b**) Placement of autologous sling under urethra, then attachment to rectus abdominus under minimal tension.

fascia. The relative risk of mesh erosion using artificial mesh has not been well published; there are no randomized trials.

HISTORICAL NOTE: STAMEY NEEDLE SUSPENSION AND RAZ/PEREYRA/GITTES PROCEDURES

In 1973, Stamey described a minimally invasive procedure to correct stress incontinence. This involved two passages of a long needle behind the pubic bone; after the first pass, a polypropylene suture was threaded through the needle. An arterial graft pledget was threaded onto the vaginal end of this suture (Figure 9.5). A second pass of the needle brought the suture back up behind the pubic bone, capturing a thick bridge of periurethral tissue; the suture was tied over the rectus sheath (then repeated

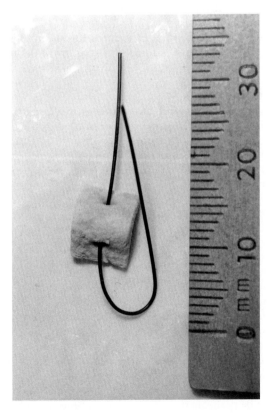

FIGURE 9.5. Stamey bladder neck suspension pledget removed from the vagina of a patient three years after the procedure.

on other side). The Raz, Pereyra, and Gittes modifications did not use the nonabsorbable pledget.

Initially the results of these procedures showed great promise, with two-year objective cure rates of 70–86% in the early 1990s (Jarvis[10]). However, over time, these cure rates were not sustained. For example, 130 patients reviewed by questionnaire at 5.5 years revealed a cure rate of 50%, but 11.5% had never become continent, 38.5% had recurrence 6–90 months after the procedure (Conrad et al[6]). Of 30 patients (interviewed and one-hour pad test) at minimum of 10 years, only 30% remained both subjectively and objectively dry (Mills et al[15]). It was thought that the pledgets/sutures had pulled through the periurethral tissue. Post-operative weight gain was associated with a higher failure rate. In a small percentage of cases, the pledget later eroded through the periurethral tissue and migrated into the vagina.

These procedures are not considered further in this text, but illustrate the importance of long-term scrutiny of the efficacy of any new surgical procedure.

PARAVAGINAL REPAIR

The paravaginal repair is often regarded as an alternative method for repair of cystocele, but has also been used to treat USI. For details, see Chapter 10 on prolapse. As regards USI, a single report showed a 97% subjective cure of stress incontinence at three- to four-year followup. Objective tests were not performed (Shull and Baden[19]).

LAPAROSCOPIC COLPOSUSPENSION

The laparoscopic colposuspension was first described in 1991. A review of 27 studies of the procedure between 1991 and 1998 ($n = 1024$) showed that only four studies used objective outcome measures, yielding a cure rate of 75% (range 60–89%) at a mean followup of 19 months (range 6–36 months, Chaliha and Stanton[5]). Only two randomized controlled trials have been published. Burton[4] showed an objective continence rate of 94% for the open Burch versus 60% for the laparoscopic Burch at three years. Tsung-Hsien Su et al[20] showed similar cure rates (96% versus 80% at one year). The risk of bladder injury in all studies was 3% (0–10%). This operation is attractive because no Pfannenstiel incision is needed, and other laparoscopic procedures can be performed at the same time. Since the advent of the TVT, use of this operation when no other laparoscopic procedures are to be performed is hard to justify, considering the expense of the equipment and questionable/unknown long-term success rates.

THE TVT AND TRANSOBTURATOR TAPE

The tension–free vaginal tape procedure has changed the management of USI. As originally designed, it is performed under local anesthetic, and most cases, can be performed as a outpatient procedure. For a registrar training in "the TVT era," it may be hard to understand just what a revolution has taken place. For 30 years (late 1960s to late 1990s), the colposuspension was the "gold standard" continence procedure. Although highly effective, it involved a five-day stay in the hospital, a 10–15% chance of detrusor overactivity, and a 2–5% chance of voiding difficulty (as above), not to mention the usual six weeks post-operative convalescence.

As outlined, the arrival of the Raz/Stamey/Peyrera/Gittes procedure brought the prospect of freedom from the Pfannenstiel incision and avoidance of prolonged convalescence. Unfortunately, these operations did not stand the test of time.

As will be shown, we now have seven- to eight-year objective data for the TVT, revealing similiar efficacy to the coloposuspension.

Pre-Operative Consent Advice

The TVT confers a 5–6% risk of detrusor overactivity, and a 1–2% risk of short-term voiding difficulty, with a 0.5% risk of long-term voiding dysfunction. Post-operatively, patients should rest for one week or until comfortable.

The TVT under local anesthesia (LA) involves the following (see Figure 9.6).

- Prepare 100 ml of LA solution, eg Prilocaine 0.25% or Naropen 0.2% with 1 ml of 1/1000 adrenaline.
- Anesthetist to give antibiotic prophylaxis against the insertion of a mesh into vaginal environment, and administer Midazolam or Propophol IV infusion for sedation.
- Empty the bladder.
- Inject LA above the pubic bone, into the retropubic space (21 gauge spinal needle), then underneath the pubic bone, then into the anterior vaginal wall, 2 cm below the urethra.
- Vertically incise the anterior vaginal wall, 2 cm below the urethra, for about 1.5 cm.
- Dissect under the vaginal skin, towards the pubic bone, left and right.

- Make a 1 cm incision at the suprapubic LA insertion sites, bilaterally.
- Insert guide wire into 16 G Foley catheter, pass into bladder.
- Assistant holds the guide/catheter to the ipsilateral side for insertion of TVT tape, to move the urethrovesical junction out of the way.
- Assemble the TVT introducer (Figure 9.6A).

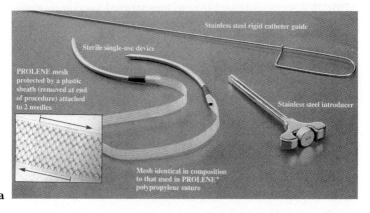

FIGURE 9.6. (a) TVT tape, guide wire, and introducer device.

- Hold edge of vaginal incision with fine Gillies forceps; insert TVT needle into incision.
- Direct needle about 30 degrees to the lateral; aim upwards towards the abdominal wound.
- Push needle firmly through the urogenital diaphragm, under strict control.
- Drop the handle of the introducer so the needle is felt to be running up the back of the pubic bone. Very gradually advance the needle up in the retropubic space until it emerges at the abdominal wound.
- Perform cystoscopy to ensure no needle puncture of bladder; empty bladder.
- Repeat procedure for the other side.
- After second cystoscopy, do not empty bladder.
- Stop IV sedation; prepare patient to cough.
- Elevate tape so it lies just under urethra (Fig. 9.6b), but insert fine scissors between tape and urethra.

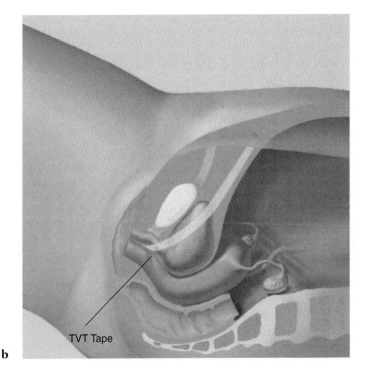

b

FIGURE 9.6. (**b**) Lateral view of TVT tape under the urethra. (Reprinted with permission from Gynecare.)

- Patient coughs repeatedly; gradually elevate the tape so that only a few drops of fluid spill over the edge of the meatus at the height of the cough (no projectile spurt).
- Assistant removes plastic covers of the tape while surgeon holds scissors to maintain tape position under the urethra (otherwise removal of the plastic tape covers can cause further elevation of the tape itself).
- Empty the bladder, close all incisions. No pack. No catheter.

Post-Operative Instructions

The patient should drink as much as she desires but not force fluids. She should void whenever she feels the desire, not at a set time. If she has not voided within four hours, bladder scan to check volume.

After each void, check residual.

If two residuals less than 100 ml, and patient comfortable, discharge home.

If residuals greater than 200, insert Foley catheter overnight; remove 6 AM; restart.

If residuals >100 ml but <200 ml, ask patient to double void and rescan; generally residuals will be less than 100 after a double void. Patient should be taught this technique.

Once patient voids completely and is comfortable, discharge.

Review at six weeks: repeat uroflowmetry/post-void ultrasound residual to check for asymptomatic voiding difficulty.

Outcome Data for the TVT

The first objective report of medium-term followup (three years) showed a dry rate on pad test of 93% (Ulmsten et al[22]). Five-year followup showed 85% objective cure rate (Nilsson et al[16]), with the same authors finding an 81% cure rate at seven years. The largest RCT (Ward and Hilton[24]) showed no significant difference between the TVT and the colposuspension at six months, and at two years (Ward and Hilton[23]).

Controversy still exists about the importance of performing the procedure under local anesthetic, and the importance of the cough test (which has also been performed under spinal or epidural anesthesia). The efficacy of TVT in the low-pressure urethra appears to be lower than in primary procedures (37–86% cure versus 88–94% cure in primary cases). For full review, see Atherton and Stanton.[2]

The risks of TVT include:

- Intra-operative perforation of bladder 4–6%
- Retropubic hematoma 2.4%
- De novo detrusor overactivity 5–6%
- Urinary tract infection 4–17%
- Short-term voiding difficulty 2–3%
- Long-term voiding dysfunction <0.5%
- From manufacturer's log of rare complications in 260,000 cases
  —Bowel perforation 0.007% (three deaths worldwide)
  —Major vascular injuries 0.012% (two deaths worldwide)
  —Urethral penetration 0.007%
  —Tape erosion 0.0013%

Some surgeons manage short-term voiding difficulty by cutting the tape; the optimum time for performing this is controversial. Continence is often preserved because the lateral arms of the tape have already become enmeshed in the periurethral tissue, providing residual support.

The Transobturator Tape

Because the TVT involves penetration of the retropubic space "blindly" (without direct vision), the above small but important risks of bowel/vascular injury are not unexpected. The Transobturator Tape was developed partly to avoid these risks, and partly to avoid the risk of penetrating the bladder in the retropubic space (thus cystoscopy is not required, and operating time is shorter). A recent report (Duval et al[7]) indicates a 90% cure rate on urodynamic testing at median follow up of 17 months.

The risk of mesh erosion is greater than TVT at 6.2%. Further long term data is needed.

THE USE OF BULKING AGENTS FOR USI

Bulking agents such as GAX collagen, macroplastique, and Durasphere are attractive because they can be performed as an out-patient procedure, have minimal risk of provoking voiding difficulty, and can be performed under local anesthesia with sedation. Unfortunately the cure rate for this procedure is variable, depending upon the agent used, the type of stress incontinence, and the number of repeat injections.

Controversy exists as to whether bulking agents should be reserved for patients with a relatively fixed bladder neck, mostly after previous continence surgery. This is probably the "standard teaching," although several trials demonstrate reasonable improvement rates in patients with a hypermobile bladder neck.

A further controversy concerns whether patients with a low urethral closure pressure (<20 cm) should be offered bulking agents. Gorton et al[8] showed clearly that the success rate over five years was significantly poorer when GAX collagen was used in women with a low urethral closure pressure. The median duration of continence for those with a low-pressure urethra was 15 months, compared to 72 months in the remainder. On Cox regression analysis, a low-pressure urethra was strongly predictive of failure ($p = 0.03$). Such data are not known for the other agents.

The procedure involves injecting approximately 4–6 ml of the bulking agent into the mid urethra, under the mucosa, via cystoscopic needle, either trans-urethrally or periurethrally, so as to "bulk up" the mid urethra (Figure 9.7).

The main features of each bulking agent are as follows.

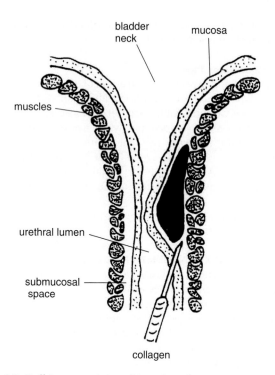

FIGURE 9.7. Bulking agent injected into the submucosa.

GAX Collagen (Contigen)
This is made of bovine dermal collagen, cross-linked with glutaraldehyde, to reduce antigenicity, first described in 1989.

- Allergic reactions to the bovine material do occur, so that skin testing is required 30 days beforehand to exclude allergic response in each patient.
- Collagen is inserted under cystoscopic control
  —Either via a trans-perineal approach, using a spinal needle, to inject periurethrally.
  —Or using a specialized cystoscopic needle, to inject trans-urethrally.
- Most surgeons inject at 6 o'clock, then 9–10 o'clock, then 2–3 o'clock.
- Each ampoule contains 2.5 ml of GAX collagen, and costs approximately 1200 Euros.

- Because bovine collagen is degraded over time, incontinence often recurs at about two years, thus "top-up" doses are commonly performed.
- Most reports of efficacy do not use objective measure.
- Khullar et al[11] showed that (on one-hour pad test) in a group of 28 elderly women (age >62, mean 76), 76% were cured at one month, falling to 48% at two years. The effect of urethral closure pressure upon success was not discussed; 16/28 had undergone previous continence surgery.

Macroplastique

This is a hydrogel-suspended cross-linked polydimethylsiloxane estomer (silicone rubber particles), first described in 1991.

- Because the particles are 100–450 microns in diameter, they do not migrate and are quickly encapsulated in fibrin.
- It is not known to produce allergic reaction.
- Initially, injection was via cystoscopic needle, trans-urethrally or trans-perineally, at 2, 6, and 10 o'clock. Each vial costs 320 pounds; two are normally used.
- In 2000, a simple applicator with specialized needle was described (see Henalla et al[13]) which avoids the need for cystoscopic visualization of the injection site (Figure 9.8). A specialized injection gun is also provided.

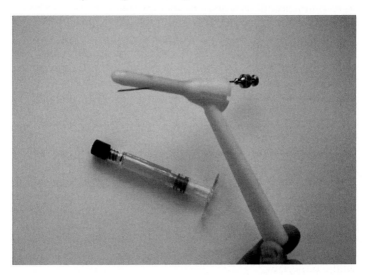

FIGURE 9.8. Macroplastique application device.

■ On subjective score, 74% of 40 women were dry at three months (Henalla et al[13]).

■ Using objective urodynamic measures, 59% of 32 women were dry at 12 months; 28 of these had undergone previous continence surgery (Koelbl et al[12]).

■ Post-operative short-term voiding difficulty and detrusor overactivity do occur with this procedure, although less commonly than for other procedures. For full review, see ter Meulen et al.[21]

Durasphere

This is a suspension of carbon-coated zirconium beads, first reported in 2001.

■ It is not known to be allergenic.

■ Using the Stamey score to grade incontinence (a nonvalidated measure), 80% of 176 women had "improvement" of at least one Stamey grade at 12 months (versus 69% of 188 women given GAX collagen; difference not significant (Lightner et al[14]). Long-term studies involving objective outcome measures are awaited.

The Cochrane review of periurethral injection therapy for urinary incontinence (Pickard et al[18]) found insufficient evidence to recommend this as a first-line therapy (implying that it should be reserved for those with previous continence surgery). None of the comparative trials revealed significant differences between the different agents in terms of efficacy. In a patient with co-morbidity that precludes anesthesia, bulking agents "may represent a useful option for relief of symptoms for a 12 month period although repeat injections are likely to be required to achieve a satisfactory result."

CONCLUSIONS

The surgical management of USI has advanced tremendously in the last two decades. Each procedure still has risks, requiring meticulous pre-operative counseling. The most appropriate procedure must be chosen for each patient, considering her previous surgical history, her willingness to undergo minimally invasive versus major surgery, and her perioperative risk factors. Careful and sympathetic management of post-operative detrusor overactivity, voiding dysfunction, and rarer complications, is vitally important.

References

1. Alcalay M, Monga A, Stanton SL (1995) Burch colposuspension: A 10–20 year followup. Br J Obstet Gynaecol 102:740–745.

2. Atherton MJ, Stanton SL (2005) The tension free vaginal tape reviewed: An evidence based review from inception to current status. Brit J Obs Gynae 112:534–546.

3. Burch JC (1968) Cooper's ligament urethrovesical suspension for stress incontinence. Am J Obs Gynecol 100:764–774.

4. Burton G (1997) A three year prospective randomised urodynamic study comparing open and laparoscopic colposuspension. Neurourol Urodyn 16:353–354.

5. Chaliha C, Stanton SL (2000) Urethral sphincter incompetence. In: Stanton SL, Monga AK eds. Clinical urogynaecology, 2nd edn., Churchill Livingstone, Harcourt, London, Chapter 19, 201–218.

6. Conrad S, Pieper A, Fernandez de la Maza S, Busch R, Huland H (1997) Long-term results of the Stamey bladder neck suspension procedure: A patient questionnaire based outcome analysis. J Urol 157:1672–1677.

7 Deval B, Ferchaux J, Berry R, Gambino S, Gofu C, Rafii A, Haab F (2006) Objective and subjective cure rates after trans-obturator tape (OBTAPE®) treatment of female urinary incontinence. European Urology 49:373–377.

8. Gorton E, Stanton S, Monga A, Wiskind AK, Lentz GM, Bland DR (1999) Periurethral collagen injection: A long-term follow-up study. Br J Urol Int 84:966–971.

9. Langer R, Rone-El R, Newman M, Herman A, Carpi D (1988) Detrusor instability following colposuspension for urinary stress incontinence. Br J Obstet Gynaecol 95:607–610.

10. Jarvis GJ (1994) Surgery for genuine stress incontinence. Br J Obstet Gynaecol 101:371–374.

11. Khullar V, Cardozo LD, Abbot D, Anders K (1997) GAX collagen in the treatment of urinary incontinence in elderly women: Two year follow up. Br J Obstet Gynaecol 104:96–99.

12. Koelbl H, Sax V, Doefler D, Haesler G, Sam C, Hanzal E (1998) Transurethral injection of silicone microimplants for intrinsic urethral sphincter deficiency. Obstet Gynecol 92:332–336.

13. Henalla SM, Hall V, Duckett JRA, Link C, Usman F, Tromaus PM et al (2000) A multicentre evaluation of a new surgical technique for urethral bulking in the treatment of genuine stress incontinence. Brit J Obstet Gynaecol 107:1035–1039.

14. Lightner DJ, Calvosa C, Andersen R (2001) A new injectable bulking agent for treatment of stress urinary incontinence: Results of a multicenter, randomized, controlled double blind study of Durasphere. Urology 58:12–15.

15. Mills R, Persad R, Handley Ashken M (1996) Long term follow up results with the Stamey operation for stress incontinence of urine. Br J Urol 77:86–88.

16. Nilsson CG, Kuuva N, Falconer C, Rezapour M, Ulmsten U (2001) Long-term results of the tension-free vaginal tape (TVT) procedure for surgical treatment of female stress urinary incontinence. Int Urogynecol J Suppl 2, S5–S8.

17. Nilsson CGN, Rezapour M, Falconer C (2003) Seven years followup of the tensions free vaginal tape procedure. Int Urogynecol J 14 (Suppl 1): S35 (abstract).

18. Pickard R, Reaper J, Wyness L, Cody DJ, McClinton S, N'Doy J (2003) Periurethral injection therapy for urinary incontinence in women. Cochrane database of systematic reviews Issue 2. CD003881. DOI: 10.1002/14651858.CD003881.

19. Shull BL, Baden WF (1989) A six year experience with paravaginal defect repair for stress urinary incontinence. Am J Obstet Gynecol 160:1432–1440.

20. Su TS, Wang KG, Hsu CY, Wei HJ, Hong BK (1997) Prospective comparison of laparoscopic and traditional colposuspension in the treatment of genuine stress incontinence. Acta Obstet Gyn Scand 76:576–582.

21. Ter Meulen PH, Berghmans LCM, van Kerrebroeck PEVA (2003) Systematic review: Efficacy of silicone microimplants (Macroplastique) therapy for stress urinary incontinence in adult women. Eur Urol 44:573–582.

22. Ulmsten U, Johnson P, Rexapour M (1999) A three year followup of tension free vaginal tape for surgical treatment of female stress urinary incontinence. Br J Obstet Gynaecol 106:345–350.

23. Ward K, Hilton P (2001) A randomised trial of colposuspension and tension-free vaginal tape (TVT) for primary genuine stress incontinence – 2 year followup. Int Urogynecol J 12 (Suppl 3):S7.

24. Ward KL, Hilton P (2002) Prospective multicentre randomised trial of thension-free tape and colposuspension as primary treatment for stress incontinence. BMJ 325:67–70.

Chapter 10
Management of Prolapse

Uterovaginal prolapse is very common. The largest epidemiological study to date (n = 1547 women interviewed, age 15–79) showed that 8.8% had symptomatic prolapse and a further 23% had undergone some form of prolapse surgery (MacLennan et al[10]).

NONSURGICAL MANAGEMENT OPTIONS

The treatment of symptomatic prolapse is largely surgical. Nevertheless, some patients attend with mild symptoms and mild prolapse, to ask whether they "need" surgery. There are no data to guide such patients. If a patient has mild asymptomatic prolapse, dealing with the precipitating factors (as per Chapter 1), along with a pelvic floor training program (Chapter 6), may be sufficient.

Use of Ring Pessary

In patients with symptomatic prolapse, who decline to have or are totally unfit for surgery, a vaginal ring pessary is very useful in selected cases. The main reasons for which patients are totally unfit for surgery are as follows.

- Multiple co-morbidities especially in the elderly.
- Severe respiratory embarrassment, unable to lie flat without dyspnea
- Transplant patients with pelvic kidney, on immunosuppressive drugs
- Severe Altzheimer's disease, unable to tolerate hospitalization
- Morbid obesity, poor surgical access to the vagina
- Unstable heart disease
- Recurrent thrombo-embolic events, multiple previous stroke

Patients may decline surgery if they are an elderly sole caregiver for an ill husband, or if they are sole caregiver for a disabled relative with no suitable respite care. Some women have had unpleasant surgical or anesthetic experiences, and do not want another surgical episode. These reasons should be respected, especially if a ring pessary can be easily fitted.

Traditional vaginal ring pessaries come in a range of sizes, from 56 mm to 100 mm diameter. Fitting a ring pessary is like assessing cervical dilatation in labor ward. Insert two fingers into the vagina, spread them apart, and mentally measure the vaginal diameter. In the United States, Gellhorn pessaries are used for large prolapse, and in the United Kingdom, shelf pessaries are also used. In Australia, the bladder neck support device is also used for severe prolapse. The ring pessary sits anteriorly behind the pubic bone, and posteriorly rests on the perineal body.

Hence if the perineum is very deficient, a ring pessary may not "sit" properly, and be extruded during defecation. In a series of 100 patients with prolapse in the United States, 73% could be fitted satisfactorily (Clemens et al[3]). A deficient perineum with large introitus was often associated with failure.

In some cases, it may be possible to overcome this by fitting a "double ring", using the largest ring possible in the upper vagina, and the next smaller ring beneath it. This will not solve the problem if the patient has had multiple previous surgeries with scarring/thickening of the walls and vaginal shortening.

Topical vaginal estrogen cream (eg Ovestin) should be used three times weekly, because the ring pessary is a foreign body which may increase desquamation of the vaginal epithelium, leading to a watery creamy discharge. It is traditional to change the ring every four to five months, to inspect the vagina to ensure no major vaginal inflammation is occurring. In a tightly fitting pessary, or when Ovestin is not used, or when the pessary is not changed regularly, there is a recognized incidence of vaginal bleeding. If this occurs, remove the ring, ask the patient to cleanse the vagina with salt baths twice daily for five to seven days, and apply Ovestin nightly for three weeks. If there is an associated purulent discharge, metronidazole 400 mg TDS for seven days will resolve this.

SURGERY FOR CYSTOCOELE

The opening paragraph of the relevant chapter in the World Health Organization monograph on incontinence states that "experts and the majority of published literature suggest the anterior wall is probably the most challenging part of prolapse to cure" (Brubaker et al[2]). This is largely because there are few structures to "anchor" on to. Unlike repair of posterior wall prolapse, in which one can suture onto the sacrospinous ligament or the presacral ligament on the sacral promontory, the pubourethral/pubocervical fascia and paravesical fascia on the undersurface of the pubic rami may be thin and weak. The main surgical options for repair of the anterior wall (also known as the "anterior compartment") comprise:

- Anterior colporrhaphy with plication of the pubourethral amd vaginal fascia
- Anterior colporrhaphy with more vigororous plication of sub-pubic fascia
- Paravaginal repair (either vaginal or abdominal approach)
- Use of mesh to reinforce the anterior colporrhaphy

Anterior Colporrhaphy

The anterior colporrhaphy for cystocele is performed as follows (see Figure 10.1).

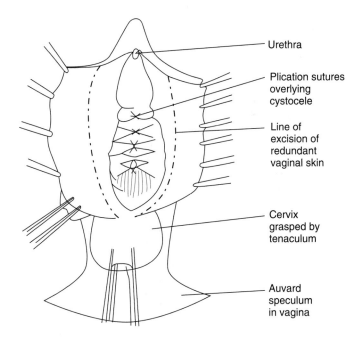

Urethra

Plication sutures overlying cystocele

Line of excision of redundant vaginal skin

Cervix grasped by tenaculum

Auvard speculum in vagina

FIGURE 10.1. Routine anterior colporrhaphy.

- Inject local anesthetic with adrenaline into subcutaneous plane of anterior wall.
- Dissect vaginal epithelium off the bladder and proximal urethra.
- Plicate the paraurethral and paravesical tissue with a sagittal tier of horizontal mattress sutures, without tension.
- Trim the redundant vaginal skin sparingly and close.
- Insert pack and suprapubic catheter.

The Anterior Repair with Extensive Plication (Ultralateral Anterior Colporrhaphy)

- The procedure starts with same dissection of vagina from bladder.
- In this case, dissect well back into the pelvis; get under the pubic symphysis.
- Place delayed–absorbable vertical mattress sutures into the pubourethral/pubocervical or paravaginal fascia that borders the levator hiatus (underneath the pubic bone) to plicate this tissue across the midline under moderate tension, thus replacing the bladder into the abdominal cavity.

Closure with trimming of vaginal skin is identical to anterior colporrhaphy.

A similar procedure involving plication of the pubourethral "ligaments" has been recommended by Nichols;[13] see Figure 10.2.

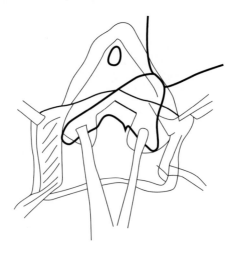

FIGURE 10.2. Plication of the pubourethral ligaments.

The recurrence rate for cystocele after routine anterior colporrhaphy is up to 40%. Few series of the more vigorous ultralateral approach have been published. The procedure remains popular because of minimal surgical morbidity.

Paravaginal Defect Repair

This has been the subject of several publications in the last two decades, but these mainly consider it as a treatment for stress incontinence, rather than for cystocele alone. Because effective operations are available for USI, but cystocele remains a difficult area, a long-term followup study of paravaginal repair for cystocele alone is urgently needed.

The paravaginal defect can be repaired trans-abdominally or vaginally. Most gynecologists would be reluctant to perform an abdominal procedure for an isolated cystocele. If cystocele co-exists with stress incontinence, then the colposuspension is highly curative of both. Therefore trans-abdominal repair of paravaginal defect is not considered further (but see Shull[14]).

The vaginal approach to paravaginal defect repair is somewhat "challenging," inasmuch as the obturatur internus muscle must be identified first by palpation and then by inspection, so the white line of the arcus tendineus fasciae pelvis can be identified. This involves use of specialized illuminated retractors, to deflect the bladder into the midline. To date, little objective outcome data has been provided to support the application of this technique.

Use of mesh to reinforce the anterior wall has received little systematic study. The first randomized controlled trial compared simple anterior repair, versus anterior repair including use of polyglactin (Vicryl) mesh, versus "ultralateral" anterior repair, in 83 patients reviewed at two years. Results (using POPQ and symptom score) revealed that 30% of the anterior repair group, 42% of the repair plus mesh, and 46% of the "ultralateral" repair patients achieved normal vaginal anatomy (POPQ stage 0 or 1). This definition of "cure" is quite strict. The authors pointed out that anterior colporrhaphy often simply does not replace the midpoint of the vagina to a level 3 cm above the introitus. Nevertheless, they concluded that the addition of mesh did not significantly improve the cure rate (Weber et al[18]).

An Italian study of polypropylene (Prolene) mesh repair for cystocele in 32 women, at a mean followup of 1.5 years, found that dyspareunia was increased by 20%; 6.5% of women had mesh erosion. Despite a 94% anatomical cure rate (using POPQ), the authors concluded that the use of prolene mesh repair of prolapse should be abandoned because of associated morbidity (Milani et al[12]). Use of similar mesh in 64 women with cystocele in Australia yielded 4.7% erosion rate, and recurrence at two years in 10% (Dwyer and O'Reilly[4]). Similar results were seen using the same mesh in 38 women from Taiwan (erosion rate 10.5%, cure 87% at two years, Hung et al[6]). All of these series varied in the selection of patients (primary versus previously failed prolapse surgeries). At present it would seem that use of mesh for a primary cystocele repair is not warranted, and use in previously failed cases requires careful discussion.

What Is the Value of Manchester Repair/Retention of a Nonprolapsed Uterus?

In a patient with a cystocele, in whom the cervix is bulky, protuberant, and somewhat elongated, without evidence of actual uterine descent, a Manchester Repair may be useful. This comprises anterior colporrhaphy with amputation of the cervix, as well as using sutures from the transverse cervical ligaments to enhance elevation of the upper vagina.

The Manchester Repair (Figure 10.3) was developed in the 1950s, at a time when anesthetic risks were greater than now. Thus a simple procedure to remove an offending organ (the bulky protuberant cervix) without the prolonged anesthesia of a vaginal hysterectomy, was attractive.

As anesthetic agents/morbidity improved, a concept evolved that if any part of the uterus/vagina was prolapsing, it should be removed/repaired. The extra time required for a vaginal hysterectomy was no longer an anesthetic issue.

In the last decade, greater scrutiny has been given to the concept of "If any part of the uterus prolapses, remove it all." A gradually increasing perception of vault prolapse has pervaded the urogynecological community. Laparoscopic procedures to suspend the uterus from the presacral ligament in cases of prolapse (laparoscopic hysteropexy) have been the subject of sporadic reports. Because no large clinical trials have been reported, this procedure is not further discussed. Nevertheless, gynecologists have perhaps appreciated that women do not want their uterus removed unless the evidence proves this will give the best result. Inasmuch as we do not know how to predict vault prolapse, a "fall-back" approach may be to leave the uterus intact unless it is truly prolapsed.

Of course the converse argument is that one is leaving a potentially malignant organ (the uterus) in situ. Furthermore, because one cannot guarantee that the cervix is completely removed, Pap smears are still required after Manchester Repair.

Nevertheless, the Manchester Repair has been used for 60 years, and is worth consideration in selected cases.

The Manchester Repair is as follows.

■ Inject local anesthetic into the anterior and posterior walls of the cervix.

■ Circumferentially incise the cervix, as for the commencement of a vaginal hysterectomy, but simply amputate the cervix (Fig. 10.3a).

■ Push up the bladder anteriorly.

■ Use curved Kocher's forceps to clamp the tranverse cervical ligaments.

■ Suture with No. 1 Vicryl and place ties on Kryal's forceps.

■ Perform a Posterior Sturmdorf suture to cover the posterior cervix with vaginal epithelium, but leave the os patent. (See Fig. 10.3b), then plicate the fransverse cervical ligaments (10.3c).

■ Carry out anterior colporrhaphy, but when closing the anterior leaves of the vaginal skin, the lower margin of the skin is again used to cover the cervix, to the level of the os.

Pre-Operative Consent Discussion for Anterior Compartment Repairs

Consent discussion involves routine discussion of mode of anesthesia to be chosen, the risks of hemorrhage, infection, and vaginal scarring. The risk of voiding difficulty is small. If anterior repair is performed in isolation, a urethral catheter may be sufficient, especially if no bladder neck buttress suture (described in Chapter 10) is needed. For patients having cystocele repair combined with other procedures, a supra-pubic catheter is usual, hence trial of void protocol should be explained. In patients having mesh inserted, risk of erosion must be explained.

Post-operative convalescence depends on whether other procedures are performed: if an isolated anterior repair, patient should rest for one week then have light duties for four weeks, and avoid heavy lifting for another four weeks.

SURGERY FOR RECTOCELE/DEFICIENT PERINEUM

Before embarking upon a "posterior repair", check whether the patient truly has

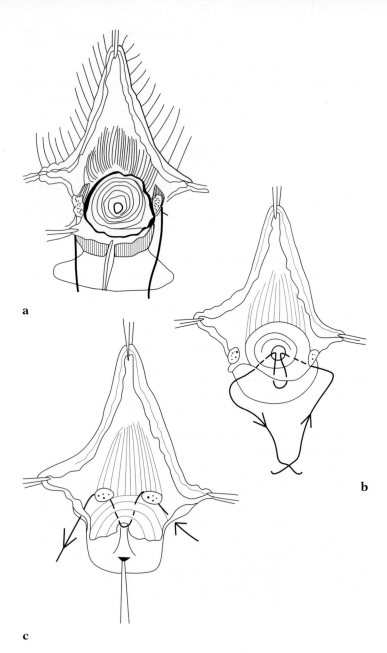

FIGURE 10.3. Posterior Sturmdorf suture in the Manchester Repair. After amputation of the cervix, seen in (a), then the posterior leaf of the vaginal vault is brought up over the posterior cervix and the Sturmdorf suture is used to fix the vault to the cervix while leaving the cervical os patent (b). The transverse cervical ligaments are then plicated (c) to facilitate elevation of the uterine body within the pelvis.

■ A deficient perineum, requiring perineorrhaphy.
■ An isolated rectocele, requiring posterior colporrhaphy, which may
　—Just involve the lower third of the rectum.
　—Or the hernia may include the mid rectum and the upper rectum.
　—The latter is often associated with enterocoele.
■ Or both of the above.

For example, in Chapter 2 (Figure 2.2b), a patient with an isolated rectocele was shown. As discussed, depending upon symptoms, she may be better served by a trans-anal repair, with no disruption of her intact perineum (Chapter 8, Figure 8.5).

Note that the deficient perineum and low rectocele is usually associated with insufficiently repaired obstetric lacerations, whereas the mid/high rectocele is often associated with constipation.

In the 1950s the standard repair of low rectocele (posterior colporrhaphy) and deficient perineum (perineorrhaphy) involved plication of the edges of the levator ani, known as "levatorplasty". In 1959, Jeffcoate[7] published a series revealing that 50–60% of patients undergoing this procedure experienced dyspareunia, especially when the levatorplasty is extended upward to repair a defect of the middle third of the rectum.

Subsequent anatomical studies revealed that the rectovaginal septum is a sheet of fibroelastic tissue between the rectum and vagina, which is often torn during parturition or repeated straining at stool. Repair of this layer does help to correct rectocele but does not cause dyspareunia. Much has been written about this subject, which is beyond the scope of this text. See Nichols and Randall[13] for full discussion.

A Repair for Mid-Low Rectocele and Deficient Perineum
■ Inject local anesthetic into the subepithelial plane of the posterior vaginal wall.
■ Decide the lateral margins of the repair.
■ The final opening should admit two or three fingers easily.
■ A midline vertical incision is made, up to the apex of the rectocele.
■ The vaginal skin is dissected off the rectovaginal septum.
　—If a low rectocele only, and levatorplasty is desired by the surgeon, dissect out as far laterally as possible, to reach the medial margins of the levator ani and the terminal ends of the bulbocavernosus and transverse perineal muscles in the lower vagina/perineum.

—The fascia of the rectovaginal septum is closed over the low rectocele using mattress sutures laterally from left to right.

—Interrupted sutures of No. 1 Vicryl are taken deeply through the medial borders of the perirectal fascia and levator ani from left to right, to tighten the muscles and fascia over the defect in the lower rectal wall (Figure 10.4).

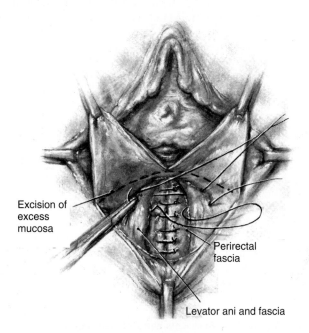

Excision of excess mucosa

Perirectal fascia

Levator ani and fascia

FIGURE 10.4. Interrupted sutures in the levator ani muscles for traditional repair of low rectocele. (Reprinted from Mattingly RF (1977) Relaxed vaginal outlet, rectocoele and enterocoele. In: Te Linde RW, Mattingl RF (eds) Te Linde's operative gynecology, 5th edn. Lippincott Williams & Wilkins, Philadelphia, p 605.)

■ The perineum is then reconstituted, by placating medial fibers
of the pubococcygeus muscles and re-uniting torn fibers of the
superficial transverse perineal muscles.
■ The redundant vaginal mucosa is excised with care.
■ The vaginal epithelium is closed.

The concept of site-specific defect repair of the rectovaginal
septum has become more widely accepted since its introduction
in the early 1990s. In brief, anatomical dissections have indicated
that lateral or "hockey-stick" shaped tears in the rectovaginal
septum (also known as the fascia of Denonvilliers) are important
in the genesis of rectocele, and that specific reconstitution of
this layer is an important part of rectocele repair. The septum
should also be re-attached to the perineal body (during its
reconstitution). For full details, see Grody.[5] Certainly in mid
and high rectocele, such site-defect repair is important.
(Figure 10.5).

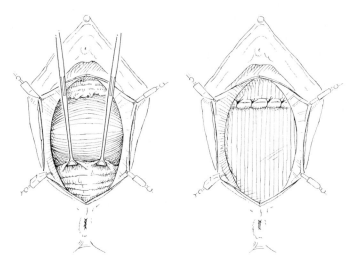

FIGURE 10.5. Example of site-specific defect repair. (Reprinted from
Grody MHT (2003) Posterior compartment defects. In: Rock JA, Jones
III HW (eds) Te Linde's operative gynecology, 9th edn. Lippincott
Williams & Wilkins, Philadelphia, p 969.)

SURGERY FOR ENTEROCELE

This is one of the most controversial areas in urogynecology. At the level of the pre-membership registrar, the question is whether to perform

- A routine posterior colporrhaphy with ligation of the enterocele sac
- A vaginal sacrospinous fixation
- An abdominal sacrocolpopexy using mesh attached to the sacrum

   The judgment as to which is best depends upon

- The frailty of the patient
- Whether the patient wishes to be sexually active
- Whether the enterocele is primary or follows previous surgery
- Whether a concomitant vaginal or abdominal procedure is required
- Whether previous vaginal repair has rendered the vaginal introitus narrow, so that a vaginal procedure would necessitate re-entry into an adequate introitus

   In a frail patient who does not wish sexual activity, posterior colporrhaphy with enterocele sac ligation is appropriate, unless this is a recurrent large enterocele, in which case sacrospinous fixation is probably necessary.

   In a fit, sexually active woman with a primary enterocele, the vaginal approach via sacrospinous fixation would be chosen by most surgeons. Others would argue that the higher long-term failure rate of the sacrospinous fixation indicates that, especially in younger women, an abdomino-sacro colpopexy should be performed. In our Unit, we would not normally undertake an abdominal incison in an active young woman, as a primary procedure. In the case of recurrent enterocele (after previous repairs, but certainly if a sacrospinous fixation has failed), abdomino-sacro colpopexy is generally chosen, unless the woman is quite elderly/frail, and prefers to have a repeat vaginal sacrospinous fixation (after appropriate counseling). The other choice in a frail woman is colpocleisis (obliteration of the vagina).

   For details of colpocleisis and enterocele sac ligation, see standard gynecology texts such as Te Linde.[16]

Vaginal Sacrospinous Fixation

This involves the following.

- Assess where the apex of the vagina will lie by grasping the apex with an Allis forceps, then reducing it into the vagina, placing it at the level of the ischial spine.

■ Leave about 2 cm of vaginal tissue intact at the apex, so as to be able to run the two pulley sutures under this segment of intact vagina (this segment will then be fastened to the sacrospinous ligament; see Figure 10.6).

■ Dissect the posterior vaginal wall, as for commencement of posterior colporrhaphy.

■ Just to the right of the midline, dissect deep into the perirectal space.

■ Gently dissect with the index finger a window in the rectal pillar, allowing one to palpate the ischial spine directly, then gradually enlarge the window to admit both index and third fingers.

■ Insert the two pulley sutures (1 nylon and 1 PDS) onto sacrospinous ligament at a point two fingerbreadths medial to the ischial spine (to avoid the pudendal nerve and vessels).

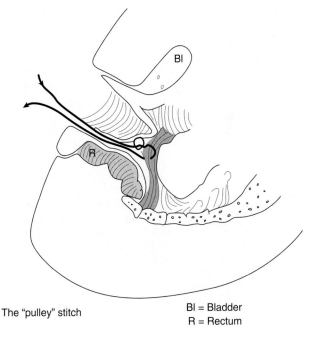

The "pulley" stitch

Bl = Bladder
R = Rectum

FIGURE 10.6. Insertion of the pulley suture to vaginal apex, and attachment to sacrospinous ligament.

Older textbooks feature suture placement under direct vision, using a Miya hook. A much simpler technique is to use a Schutt arthroscopic needle holder (also called a Caspari needle holder) shown in Figure 10.7; the thread is fed through the

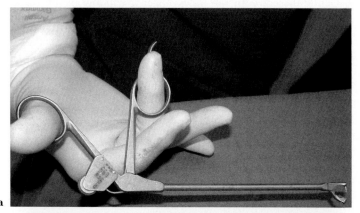

a

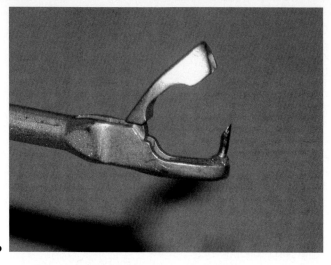

b

FIGURE 10.7. (a) and (b) Arthroscopic needle holder (manufactured by Zimmer). With closeup of open jaws that encircle the sacrospinous ligament.

device and caught between the two fingers as it emerges from the ligament.

■ Before tying down the pulley sutures, commence closure of the apex vaginal skin for about 3 cm (this section will become inaccessible once the pulley sutures are tied down).

■ Also, ensure that rectovaginal septum repair sutures or levatorplasty sutures have been inserted appropriately and held out of the way of the pulley sutures.

■ After tying down the pulley sutures, tie off the mid or low rectocele repair sutures, then complete closure of posterior vaginal mucosa.

■ At the perineum, insert appropriate perineorrhaphy sutures before closing perineal skin.

■ Insert vaginal pack, suprapubic catheter.

Pre-Operative Consent Discussion for Vaginal Sacrospinous Fixation

Consent discussion involves the following.

Risk of buttock pain 6% (chronic 1%)
Risk of de novo stress incontinence 2.6%
Risk of de novo dyspareunia 2.7%
Risk of de novo fecal incontinence 4%
Risk of de novo cystocele 8% (if no concomitant anterior repair)

These risks are derived from 293 cases (Lovatsis and Drutz[9]). The success of the procedure is variable depending upon method of assessment, eg 88% success at six weeks on strict anatomical criteria (no prolapse below the mid vagina[15]) or 97% at one year (symptomatic prolapse, or an asymptomatic prolapse at or beyond the introitus[9]).

Because many patients having a sacrospinous fixation also require other procedures, we find it helpful to draw a diagram of the anatomical defects (see Figure 10.8A for a patient with enterocele, rectocele, and cystocele) and then superimpose an outline of the surgical procedures on this diagram (see Figure 10.8B for a patient undergoing sacrospinous fixation with anterior and posterior repair).

Abdominal Sacro-Colpopexy

This involves the following.

■ A Pfannenstiel or vertical midline incision (depending on previous scars and obesity).

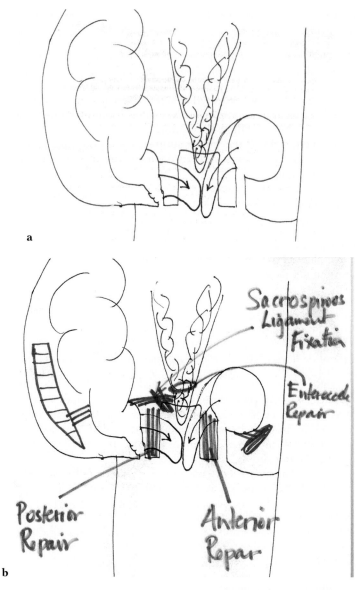

FIGURE 10.8. (a) Diagram of the anatomical defects for a patient with enterocele, rectocele, and cystocele. (b) Outline of the surgical procedures for a patient undergoing sacrospinous fixation with anterior and posterior repair.

- The vagina is elevated with a probe wrapped in gauze.
- The peritoneum over the vaginal vault is incised, abdominally.
- The bladder is reflected forward from the anterior vaginal wall.
- The peritoneum is entered in the pouch of Douglas.
- The rectum is deflected to the left, so that the peritoneal incision is extended up along the right paracolic gutter towards the sacral promontory.
- The peritoneum over the sacral promontory is carefully incised and spread open, taking care not to injure the presacral vessels.
- A wide-pore mesh such as Vipro-II is fashioned into a Y-shape by the surgeon (Figure 10.9).
- The bottom of the Y (both leaves) is attached over the apex of the vagina with nonabsorbable sutures.
- The top single leaf of the Y is run laterally up to the pre-sacral ligament over S1.
- It is attached to the ligament by nonabsorbable sutures.
- The peritoneum is closed over the mesh entirely.
- The pouch of Douglas is closed to prevent further enterocele, by a Moscovitch or Halban's procedure.
  - —The Moscovitch procedure involves a spiral suture around the edges of the pouch of Douglas to close it circumferentially.
  - —The Halban's procedure involves a series of left to right sutures in the sagittal plane that close the anterior and posterior leaves of the pouch of Douglas.
- The pouch of Douglas is drained.
- At end of abdominal procedure, assess the lower vagina.
  - —A low cystocele may indicate anterior repair.
  - —A low rectocele or deficient perineum may indicate colporrhaphy or perineorrhaphy.
  - —Vaginal pack and choice of catheter depending upon whether low vaginal procedures were undertaken.

Pre-Operative Consent Discussion for Abdomino-Sacrocolpopexy
Consent discussion involves the following.

- If the patient has a need to digitate to evacuate the stool preoperatively, that may persist in up to half of the cases (Baessler and Schuessler[1] $n = 33$).
- Careful management of constipation (Chapters 6 and 8) must be undertaken preoperatively.
- Complications (from Valaitis and Stanton[17] $n = 41$) include
  - —New or worsened detrusor overactivity (7%).

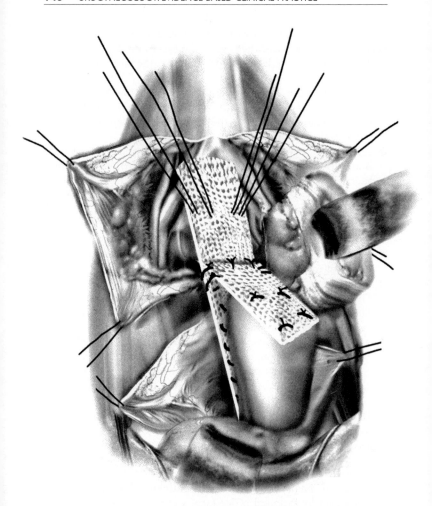

FIGURE 10.9. Y-shaped mesh inserted over the vaginal vault, the long end of the "Y" is attached to the pre-sacral ligament. (Reprinted with permission from Baggish MS, Karram MM (2001) Atlas of pelvic anatomy and gynaecological surgery, p 280. Copyright 2001, Elsevier.)

—New or worsened stress incontinence (12.5%).
—Dyspareunia (9.7%).
■ The success rate varies from 88% at two years (Valaitis and Stanton[17]) to 100% cure of enterocele at two years but persistent rectocele in 48% (Baessler and Schuessler[1] this picture is

quite complex as not all pre-operative rectoceles were corrected).

The Cochrane review concluded that abdominal sacro-colpopexy conferred a lower rate of recurrent prolapse versus vaginal sacrospinous fixation (relative risk 0.23, 95% CI 0.07–0.77) and less dyspareunia, but the vaginal procedure was quicker, cheaper, and allowed earlier return to activities of daily living (Maher et al[11]).

Note: The subject of uterine prolapse is dealt with in standard gynecological textbooks, and is not discussed here. If the uterus prolapses to the mid vagina, then vaginal hysterectomy is generally indicated, which may be a part of any of the procedures in this chapter. Procedures to suspend the vault (McCaull's culdoplasty etc) should always be considered. If the uterus descends within the upper vagina, the decision for removal should be based upon gynecological considerations (menorrhagia etc), tempered by a discussion of the patient's wishes. The option of Manchester repair has been described.

CONCLUSIONS

The average life span of women in the Western world is currently about 80 years, and is gradually increasing. Hence prolapse is likely to increase. Although the last two decades have shown improved techniques in the management of prolapse, the Cochrane Collaboration criticizes a serious lack of randomized controlled trials of new interventions. Several procedures have been mentioned only briefly in this chapter because little objective data were available. It is hoped that in the next decade more objective studies including comparative results will be published.

References

1. Baessler K, Schuessler B (2001) Abdomino sacro colpopexy and anatomy and function of the posterior compartment. Obstet Gynecol 97:678–684.
2. Brubaker L, Bump R, Jacquetin B, Schuessler B, Weidner A, Zimmern P, Milani R (2002) Pelvic organ prolapse. In: Abrams P, Cardozo L, Khoury S, Wein A (eds) Incontinence, Second International Consultation on Incontinence. Health Publication, Plymbridge Distributors, Plymouth UK, Chapter 5, pp 243–266.
3. Clemens JL, Aguilar VC, Tillinghast TA, Jackson ND, Myers DL (2003) Risk factors associated with an unsuccessful pessary fitting trial in women with pelvic organ prolapse. Neurourol Urodyn 22:648–653.

4. Dwyer PL, O'Reilly BA (2004) Trans vaginal repair of anterior and posterior compartment with Atrium polypropylene mesh. Brit J Obstets Gynaecol 111:831–836.
5. Grody MHT (2003) Posterior compartment defects. In: Rock JA, Jones HW (eds) Te Linde's operative gynecology 9th edn. Lippincott William & Wilkins, Philadelphia, pp 966–985.
6. Hung, MJ, Liu FS, Shen et al (2004) Factors that affect recurrence after anterior colporrhaphy procedure reinforced with four-corn anchored polypropylene mesh. Int Urogynecol J 15:399–400.
7. Jeffcoate TNA (1959) Posterior colporrhaphy. Am J Obstet Gynecol 77:490.
8. Kohli N, Sze EHM, Roat TW, Karram MM (1996) Incidence of recurrent cystocoele after anterior colporrhaphy with and without concomitant transvaginal needle suspension. Am J Obstet Gynecol 175:1476–1482.
9. Lovatsis D, Drutz HP (2002) Safety and efficacy of sacrospinous vault suspension. Int Urogynecol J 13:308–313.
10. MacLennan AH, Taylor AW, Wilson DH, Wilson D (2000) The prevalence of pelvic floor disorders and their relationship to gender, age, parity and mode of delivery. Br J Obstet Gynaecol 107:1460–1470.
11. Maher C, Baessler K, Glazener CMA, Adams EJ, Hagen S (2004) Surgical management of pelvic organ prolapse in women. Cochrane Library, Issue 4, Article number CD004014.pub2.
12. Milani R, Salvatore S, Soligo M, Pifarotti P, Meschia M, Cortese M (2005) Functional and anatomical outcome of anterior and posterior vaginal prolapse repair with prolene mesh. BJOG 112:107–111.
13. Nichols DH, Randall CL (1996) Vaginal surgery 4th edn. Williams and Wilkins, Baltimore, pp 258–283.
14. Shull B (2003) Paravaginal defect repair; Surgical correction of defects in pelvic support. In: Rock JA, Jones HW (eds) Te Linde's operative gynecology 9th edn. Lippincott William & Wilkins, Philadelphia, Chapter 35, pp 957–962.
15. Shull BL, Capen CV, Riggs MW, Kuehl TJ (1992) Preoperative and postoperative analysis of site-specific pelvic support defects in 81 women treated with sacrospinous ligament suspension and pelvic reconstruction. Am J Obstet Gynecol 166:1764–1171.
16. Te Linde's operative gynaecology (2003) 9th edn. Lippincott Williams and Wilkins, Philadelphia.
17. Valaitis SR, Stanton SL (1994) Sacrocolpopexy: a retrospecture study of a clinician's experience. Br J Obstets and Gynaecol 101:518–522.
18. Weber AM, Walter MD (1997) Anterior vaginal prolapse: Review of anatomy and techniques of surgical repair. Obstet Gynecol 89:311–318.
19. Weber AM, Walters MD, Piedmaont MR, Ballard LA (2001) Anterior colporrhaphy: A randomized trial of three surgical techniques. Am J Obstet Gynecol 185:1299–1304.

Chapter 11
Recurrent Bacterial Cystitis in Women

Recurrent bacterial cystitis is defined as recurrent significant bacteriuria (more than 10^5 organisms per ml of a single organism, with significant pyuria (more than 10 white blood cells per ml), in the absence of upper tract pathology. "Recurrent" is usually taken to mean more than three proven UTIs in the last five years. (Because the abbreviation RBC usually applies to red blood cells, "UTI" is used here.) If upper urinary tract disorders are causing the UTI, then referral to a urologist is required. Also, if there is no upper tract disorder, but the patient has recurrent bouts of hematuria associated with the UTI, then urology referral is also indicated. Recurrent UTI is common in urogynecological patients. About 4% of women age 15–65 have significant bacteriuria at any given time (Kass et al[3]), and the prevalence rises with age. About 25% of women experience at least one proven recurrence within six months of the first attack.

GUIDE TO MANAGEMENT OF RECURRENT UTI
At the first visit, take history of "recurrent" carefully.

Obtain old MSU results from GP if possible.
Check whether the patient has episodes of multi-resistant organisms, which may explain why "recurrences" (the treatment may have been incorrect).
Check for unusual bacteria such as Proteus Mirabalis, Pseudomonas, Strep faecalis etc that may suggest upper tract disease.
Ascertain whether UTI are mainly triggered by intercourse.
Check whether previous colposuspension may have caused voiding dysfunction/high residual urine volumes.

During Examination
Check for a large cystocele that may harbor a stagnant pool of urine.

Check for atrophic vaginitis, which increases susceptibility to UTI.

INVESTIGATIONS FOR RECURRENT UTI

We find it useful to give the patient three sterile urine culture jars, and ask her to give a specimen of urine at the very first symptom of any infection, to check organism type. Although dip-stick testing is cost-effective in general practice, in the patient with recurrent UTI and incontinence/prolapse, the organisms should be identified on culture. Ask for all organisms to be reported, even if count only 10^2 per ml, with pyuria.

Order a renal ultrasound and post-void residual to exclude:

- Renal calculi or pyelonephritis/hydronephrosis
- Large complex renal cysts (small simple cysts seldom warrant concern)
- Narrow mouth bladder diverticulum that may collect stagnant pool of urine
- Dilated ureters that may suggest vesicoureteric reflux (if so, order micturating cystourethrogram)

The above conditions also indicate referral to a urologist. Urine flow rate may show a picture of obstruction, suggesting urethral stenosis. Post-void ultrasound may show incomplete emptying, i.e. residual greater than 50–100 ml.

TREATMENT

If post-menopausal, treat with topical vaginal estrogen. A large RCT showed significant reduction in the incidence of UTI after estrogen versus placebo (Raz and Stamm[6]).

If post-coital UTI, we advise patients to read and practice the self-help regime of Kilmartin,[4] which contains many helpful points about pre- and post-coital techniques to reduce the risk of this distressing problem. If these techniques do not prevent recurrence, then post-coital antibiotic therapy with trimethoprim 300 mg stat or nitrofurantoin 100 mg are of proven value.

If associated with large prolapse and residual urine, consider using a vaginal ring pessary to elevate the prolapse. If this eradicates the UTI, then repair of the prolapse should be considered (even if otherwise asymptomatic). If associated with persistent residual urine volumes >50 ml (but no prolapse), teach the technique of double emptying (see Chapter 9, management of voiding difficulty).

In the nonincontinent woman, bacteriuria without pyuria is not usually treated, because it spontaneously resolves. In the incontinent woman who has frequency and urgency, we generally treat, because bacteriological studies have shown that the endotoxins produced by bacteria can reduce the contractile strength of the urethral sphincter, or decrease the contractility threshold of the detrusor, thus promoting incontinence (Moore et al[5]).

At Second Visit

If further proven UTI, consider three months of nitrofurantoin, trimethoprim therapy, or cystoscopy. These antibiotics are preferred because they are not well absorbed into the blood stream, not broad spectrum, and are not likely to cause thrush. At least three months therapy is chosen, to completely eradicate "microbiological communities" that may form within the epithelium and lamina propria of the bladder. If the patient takes three months of such therapy, and still has "break-through" UTI, then cystoscopy is indicated.

What to Look for on Cystoscopy

Exclude narrow mouthed diverticulum. One also may see small waxy-yellow raised areas of micro-abscesses, as part of "cystitis cystica" appearance. Diathermy will eradicate these.

References

1. Boos K (2001) Cystitis and urethritis. In: Cardozo L, Staskin D (eds) Textbook of female urology and urogynaecology. Martin Dunitz, London, Chapter 67, pp 866–900.
2. Foxman B (1990) Recurring urinary tract infection: Incidence and risk factors. Am J Public Health 80:331–333.
3. Kass EH, Savage W, Santamarina BAG (1965) The significance of bacteriuria in preventive medicine. In: Kass EH (ed) Progress in pyelonephritis. FA Davis, Philadelphia, pp 3–10.
4. Kilmartin A (2002) The patient's encyclopaedia of urinary tract infection, sexual cystitis and interstitial cystitis. New Century Press, Chula Vista, California.
5. Moore KH, Simons A, Mukerjee C, Lynch W (2002) Relative incidence of detrusor instability and bacterial cystitis found on the urodynamic test day. Br J Urol 85:786–792.
6. Raz R, Stamm WE (1993) A controlled trial of intravaginal estriol in post menopausal women with recurrent urinary tract infections. N Eng J Med 329:753–756.

Chapter 12
Interstitial Cystitis

Unlike the other conditions considered in this text which are very common, interstitial cystitis (IC) is quite rare. This chapter is a short summary of a great deal of research and clinical studies that have been directed at this fascinating problem. Appropriate textbooks are recommended.

HOW TO DIAGNOSE IT
IC is a chronic pain syndrome characterized by the following.

Recurrent episodes of suprapubic pain/pelvic pain.
Pain is worse when the bladder is full.
The symptom of urgency is actually painful (in 92% of cases).
Severe frequency (can void 60 times per day or more).
Generally, severe nocturia (10 times per night or more, in 51% of cases).
Leakage of urine is not typical (but can occur).

Less common symptoms include the following.

Chronic pelvic pain or pressure symptoms (64–69%)
Dysuria (61%)
Dyspareunia (55%)
Pain for days after sexual intercourse (37%)
Hematuria (22%)

IC is more common in women (ratio 9:1).

Large studies indicate prevalence of about 18 per 100,000 women (Ho et al[3]).
The annual estimated incidence is 2.6 per 100,000 total U.S. population.
The average IC patient sees three or four urologists or gynecologists before diagnosis.

The diagnosis of IC is based on:

The classic symptoms of pain with frequency/urgency/nocturia.
The Frequency Volume Chart (FVC) shows severe frequency/
nocturia.
FVC usually shows small volumes/small bladder capacity.
Urodynamic testing is painful and just shows small bladder capacity (although in some cases detrusor contractions are seen).
Voiding function is usually normal (flow rate and residual urine).
Urine cultures are generally sterile (by definition must be sterile for three months).
Cystoscopy must be performed under general anesthesia (GA).

- Mucosa often fairly normal during first fill.
- Capacity under GA is reduced, eg 400–600 ml.
- Refill exam must be performed: shows petechial hemorrhages; small punctate red dots scattered over the mucosa.
- In severe cases, may see Hunners ulcers—red splits or cracks in the mucosa.
- Bladder biopsy is recommended.

Biopsy needs special stains for mast cells (see Figure 12.1).
Often but not always reveals excess mast cells in the detrusor muscle.

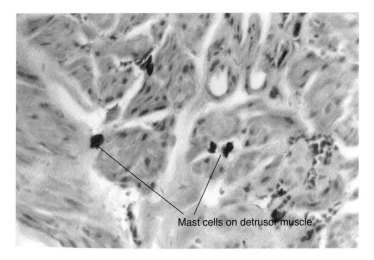

Mast cells on detrusor muscle

FIGURE 12.1. Mast cells in the detrusor muscle from a biopsy taken from patient with classic features of IC.

ETIOLOGY

The etiology of IC remains unknown, although several theories have been put forward.

The defective epithelial barrier theory: The bladder mucosa is lined by a chemical layer of glycosaminoglycans (GAGs) which are thought to render the urothelium impermeable to harmful solutes (such as urea). Early histological studies suggested that the urothelium of IC patients was more readily penetrated, but later functional radio-isotope studies showed no significant differences between IC patients and controls.

The detrusor mastocytosis theory: Because mast cells release histamine, which causes pain, hyperemia, and fibrosis, an excess of mast cells in the detrusor muscle could explain the pathophysiology of IC. An early study of 115 IC patients suggested that a finding of >28 mast cells per mm^2 in the detrusor muscle (on biopsy) indicated "true" IC and a lower mast cell count indicated early disease. Although this basic concept is still probably true, high mast cell counts can be seen in patients with prostate cancer, so the finding is not pathognomonic. Later studies showed that high mast cell counts in the lamina propria are also a marker of "classic IC". For review, see Theoharides et al, 2001.

The autoimmune theory: Several studies have shown that patients with severe IC are more likely to have antinuclear antibodies. Thus IC has been likened to scleroderma (fibrosis) but the data are inconsistent. Co-existence of IC with Sjogren's disease, rheumatoid arthritis, SLE, and Hashimoto's thyroiditis has been reported in large prevalence studies.

In the United States, the National Institute of Diabetes and Digestive and Kidney Diseases (NIDDK), which is part of the National Institutes of Health (NIH) has a major interest in funding research into IC. The NIDDK has established a national database of patients with IC, to study the long-term natural history of the disease. So far as we know at present, IC tends to wax and wane over time, but is not "curable."

TREATMENT

Cystodistension is often performed as part of the initial cystoscopy. Up to 60% of patients obtain benefit for three to six months.

Dimethyl sulfoxide (DMSO) installation is usually first-line therapy, and is the only intravesical treatment approved by the FDA in the United States. After catheterization, a 50 ml solution of DMSO is instilled into the bladder; the patient is encouraged to retain it for 15–30 minutes. Weekly or biweekly treatments are given for six to eight weeks. Response is usually noted after three to four weeks. An initial worsening of symptoms for one to two weeks may occur. A garliclike taste and skin odor are often noted for up to three days. Marked reduction in pain and frequency occur in 50–90% of patients; relapse occurs in about 40% but repeat treatment is usually effective. The drug is cheap and has no major side effects.

Amitriptyline, 25–75 mg daily, is useful in patients who can tolerate its sedative effects, with major benefit in 70–80% in such cases.

Pentosan polysulfate sodium (Elmiron) is an expensive oral drug, 100 mg TDS, for at least six months. Clinical improvement may not start until after two to four months, so therapy is recommended for six months. In open trials, up to 80% of patients note 80% reduction in pain. In placebo controlled RCTs, the drug has about double the effect of placebo (32% versus 16% objective benefit; see Pontari and Hanno[6] for review, but also Nordling.[5]

Trans-cutaneous nerve stimulation (TENS) has been used successfully to inhibit the perception of suprapubic pain. The electrodes are placed suprapubically, the stimulus is 10 Hertz, in keeping with other chronic pain therapy (see Chapter 7 for methodology).

Oxalate free diet has been used with some success. Patients avoid acidic foods such as tomatoes, strawberries, chilies, citrus fruits, tea, coffee, vinegar, and alcohol. A further modification of this diet involves avoiding foods high in tyrosine, tyramine, tryptophan, aspartate, and phenylalanine. Several studies show substantial benefit (Gillespie[1]).

Surgical resection of Hunner's ulcers by endoscopic resectoscope was originally practiced, but other treatments have superseded this because of the risk of postoperative scarring, fibrosis, and reduction of bladder capacity.

Clam Cystoplasty, as described for refractory detrusor overactivity (Chapter 7), is a useful procedure to enlarge bladder capacity and reduce pain, but has major morbidity.

Continent diversion can be used in end-stage disease (for review see Hohenfellner et al[4]).

The NIDDK operates a useful Web site for patient information; a very good leaflet can be downloaded: http://www.niddk.

nih.gov/health/urolog/pubs/cystitis/cystitis.htm. In the United States an IC patient support group is run, with a useful newsletter that is available worldwide; details at www.ichelp.org.

References

1. Gillespie L (1997) Interstitial cystitis and diet. In: Sant GR (ed) Interstitial cystitis. Lippincott-Raven, Philadelphia, Chapter 13, pp 109–115.
2. Hanno PM, Staskin Dr, Krane RJ, Wein AJ (1990) Interstitial cystitis. Springer Verlag, London.
3. Ho N, Koziol JA, Parsons CL (1997) Epidemiology of Interstitial Cystitis. In: Sant GR (ed) Interstitial Cystitis. Lippincott-Raven, Philadelphia, Chapter 2, pp 9–16.
4. Hohenfellner M, Linn J, Hampel C, Thuroff JW (1997) Surgical treatment of interstitial cystitis. In: Sant GR (ed) Interstitial cystitis. Lippincott-Raven, Philadelphia, Chapter 28, pp 223–233.
5. Nordling I (2004) Interstitial Cystitis: how should we diagnose it and treat it in 2004? Curr Opinion Urol 14:323–327.
6. Pontari MA, Hanno PM (1997) Oral therapies for interstitial cystitis. In: Sant GR (ed) Interstitial cystitis. Lippincott-Raven, Philadelphia, Chapter 22, pp 173–176.
7. Theoharides TC, Kempuraj D, Sant GR (2001) Mast cell involvement in interstitial cystitis: a seeker of human & experimental evidence. Urology 57:47–55.

Index

Page numbers followed by f indicate figures.

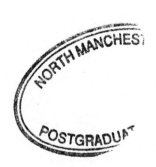